MW01254342

FINDING BALANCE

Origins: A Massage Therapist's Personal
Journey to Unlocking the Source of Your Pain

Deborah Pfingstl, RMT

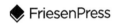 FriesenPress

One Printers Way
Altona, MB R0G 0B0
Canada

www.friesenpress.com

ISBN
978-1-03-911408-1 (Hardcover)
978-1-03-911407-4 (Paperback)
978-1-03-911409-8 (eBook)

1. HEALTH & FITNESS, EXERCISE, STRETCHING

Distributed to the trade by The Ingram Book Company

Ken

In Loving Memory of Margaret Stevens,
Peter Redman and John Redman.

Thank you for being
such an amazing friend

Well Wishes
DEffingptl

This book is dedicated to my family, clients and friends. Some are synonymous. Clients who are friends have become family, and family who are friends have become clients.

TABLE OF CONTENTS

PREFACE

One Massage Therapist's Journey

There are probably about a million massage therapists in the world and for each and every single one there is a unique style. All our life's experiences and viewpoints of the amazing human body makes each massage special. Our personal interests, our goals and training that continues after college is what molds each of us and our craft. What we choose to take from these experiences and what we choose to omit are what makes each massage unique.

This is just one massage therapist's story, mine.

INTRODUCTION

Massage therapy just came naturally to me. At the age of four I started massaging family. Later, it was friends. Eventually, I graduated to pulling neighbours out of their yards. Only the obviously injured ones of course! But it never occurred to me to do massage for a living until my 30th birthday. After 10 years working for a bank, I realized it was not what I wanted to do for the rest of my life. Sitting in a cubicle under florescent lights, high-pressure sales and stressful goal setting deadlines was not for me. I had to think about what I was good at. Let's see, I thought. There's cribbage. I could do the senior legion circuit and win some of their pension money, which would bother me considerably and I wouldn't be able to sleep at night, or I could go back to school and study massage therapy.

I was on the fence for a while about going back to school because when I was in grade nine, I knew for certain that I did not learn the same way as the other students. My reading skills were poor, which meant I had to work three times harder than everyone else to get good grades. There was no testing for dyslexia back then, but that was what it was. However, with dyslexia you are also given gifts. I was able to memorize entire paragraphs if each was written in a different colour. By the time grade twelve came along I had discovered boys, and my grades plummeted! I received a 49% in math, but they bumped me up to a 50% to pass me. Talk about graduating by the skin of your teeth! So, you can see how daunting the idea of going back to school was. If I made the change, I knew I would have to dedicate my life to it. I applied as a mature student but thought I wouldn't be accepted into college because my high school grades had been so low.

Even before I was accepted into massage therapy college, I went out and purchased two colouring books, one for anatomy and one for physiology. I had always wanted to study these subjects, but they weren't offered in high school. I knew I would have to work hard, so I began working on them with the hope of get a head start. As I mentioned above, writing each paragraph in a different coloured ink in high school was one of the ways I was able to retain information. It felt a bit like cheating, but I needed all the help I could get. The colouring books helped me memorize the body part and its function with its name, if they were all the same colour.

In 2000, I was accepted. I loved college and realized I was a complete nerd! I went from barely passing high school to pulling down 90s and 100s on my exams. I just ate it up. Yes, I had to work extra hard, but I was used to that and dove right in. I read five hours a day, every day. I needed to understand what the origin of every word was and how the body worked, right down to the molecules. Visual learning was my favorite. Gross anatomy with "muscle men" cadavers at the University of Saskatchewan medical laboratories was fascinating to me. The 3D visual of the human body with muscle layers, tissue directions, and attachments made sense to me immediately. I could now see the inside of the body and imagine the movements in my head.

My initial goal when I began college was to move to Phoenix, Arizona after graduation, where a lot of seniors go to retire. My dad and his dual-citizen wife lived in Hawaii but had a lot of friends who lived in Phoenix and could sponsor me to work there. It would have been a great opportunity and close enough for me to fly to Hawaii on weekends and help Dad in his retirement years. Unfortunately, Dad had passed away from lung cancer in my first year of college.

CHAPTER ONE

Confessions of a Massage Therapist

I've had an affinity for seniors all my life. Growing up I didn't get to know any of my grandparents and really felt like I was missing out on that part of my life. At the age of fifteen, I read in the newspaper about some Girl Scouts who were "adopting" grandparents at personal care homes. There was a personal care home not far from my home. Holding the newspaper clipping in my hand, I walked over and spoke with the ladies in the office. I hoped they would let me adopt a grandparent, even if I wasn't a Girl Scout. We sat and talked for a while, and they told me that a husband and wife had just been admitted that day and asked if I would like to meet them.

I was nervous and thrilled at the same time. I hoped they would like me and would be okay with me "adopting" them. That day, we went to their room, and the woman from the admin office explained why we were there. They sat on their beds and listened very carefully to my story. We chatted and visited for about half an hour before I nervously asked them if it would be okay for me to adopt them both. They were so sweet and kind and said 'yes.' I gave them each a hug, thanked them and told them I'd be back. When I arrived the following day, my "grandma" came to the door and invited me in. I asked where her husband was, and she told me he had passed away during the night. She was alone now, and it seemed like divine intervention to me that we had been placed together.

We spent a lot of time together. She told me amazing stories of her life and childhood. She and her mother had tickets to come to North America from England on the Titanic! Something told her not to get on the ship, and she begged her mother to not go. Fortunately, her mother listened to her. Even though the tickets must have cost a small fortune at that time, they never got on the ship. She still had the tickets they were supposed to use for their journey west on the Titanic. Our visits were many times a week and I got to know some of the other residents there as well. Saying hello and touching someone on their shoulder was a simple thing to do, but it seemed to change some of their days completely. It was an incredible feeling to know you made someone's day a bit better.

In June of the year I turned sixteen, I went to Hawaii to visit my father and his wife who had recently moved there to start a flower farm. When I returned home, my mother sat me down and explained that my grandma had passed away while I was gone. She had left me a little keepsake box that she loved with her favorite blue pin-on flower brooch inside it. My mother tucked the obituary clipping from the paper into the box as well. My heart was broken but I took my love of her and my experiences with her and the personal care home with me.

During college, I focused most of my outreach programs on working with the elderly and adults with disabilities. I loved it. My heart was still in it and it became a part of my drive during my college years. In school, we'd had one therapist who spoke about working with the elderly, so after college I contacted her for advice about how to get started. At the same time, I got a seniors housing guide from the Age and Opportunity Foundation and started making cold calls to their assisted-living facilities. I asked their social workers if I could come in and give massage therapy presentations. Most of them were very interested and willing to let me come in to speak. I did presentation after presentation for months at these residences. Most seniors' exposure to massage therapy was little to none. For many, the practice wasn't a part of their cultures when they were growing up. The practice, as a healing technique, only became accepted in Canada about 40 years prior.

It was a tough slog getting these hesitant folks to try massage, but usually, when one brave soul did, many others stepped forward. It wasn't an overnight success by any means. I had to earn my salt every single day. The words of my instructors kept running through my head. "Respect takes a long time to achieve but one second to lose." I promised myself that I would always try to treat these kind people with the respect I would have wanted others to show to my father or grandma. I was fortunate to meet some incredibly open-minded and patient people, one of which whom is still with me, nineteen years later!

I really got my feet wet working as a mobile massage therapist with people who'd had strokes or arthritis, or both. Once a week I held a paraffin wax therapy day at one of my assisted living buildings. This wax has mineral oils in it to help it melt at a lower temperature, so no one gets burned. The mineral oil in the wax is also great for the skin, making it soft and pliable. The moist heat from the wax penetrates the joints and stimulates the synovial fluids, which act like lubricant inside the joint capsules. We had fun and began to see positive changes.

Sweet little old ladies with gnarly crooked fingers would come down to the hairdressing room where I set up during times it was not being used as a hair salon. The wax was an excellent tool to use for arthritis. We would coat their arthritic hands or feet with the wax and wrap them in plastic. An oven mitt or towel would insulate the heat. If someone had an arthritic shoulder or knee, I would use a paintbrush to apply the wax to that area. It was a huge success! Fingers began to straighten after just a few treatments! Knees the size of large grapefruits were going down to normal size! Pain medications were reduced or no longer needed for some of these people. This therapy was so successful that my clients got better and didn't need me anymore. One lady loved the paraffin wax so much she bought her own kit. I kept one day a week for my mobile massage clients. Some stuck with me for years and some for over a decade.

In 2004, after two years working as a mobile massage therapist and learning with my seniors in assisted living, it was time for me to try working in personal care homes. They say when you are on the right path in life things come easy. There were three personal care homes close to where I lived that I was interested in working at, so I pitched my idea to each of them. They all bought it! For over ten years, I had the extreme pleasure and honour to work with the elderly and disabled adults who resided in these personal care homes. They taught me so much, things you just can't learn in school. You would expect them to be depressed or miserable in these places, but they surprised me! Don't get me wrong, there were some depressed and cranky folks there, but the majority taught me how to love each day and laugh at it. I admired their grace in the face of death.

Despite their incredible injuries these amazing people found a way to do everything and by that, I mean everything! I quickly learned to knock before I entered a room. They aren't always sleeping… One day I found a man and a woman, completely naked, going at it on the floor and both obviously enjoying themselves. He had gotten out of his wheelchair, and she out of her bed, and they were fully undressed. There are some things you just can't *un-see*. I am not a prude. These are people with natural people needs. It's a healthy normal part of life. There were conjugal visits from wives and husbands all the time, and since there was no scarf or handkerchief hanging on the doorknobs, you stopped and thought twice when you saw a closed door.

We like to think about these adorable grannies and grandpas as sweet innocent people all their lives. PAH! During the depression some of these people were getting high smoking beet leaves. Where there's a will there's a way. There were hidden mickeys of whatever tucked into plant pots. These weren't dying people; these were dorm rooms!

Being a person in a position of trust I got to hear all their wild stories. Fortunately for you, I am bound by confidentiality and won't share all the gory details. I can say one such story involved a resident giving a Handi-Transit driver a blow job! She described it down to the colour of his long johns. Needless to say, there are somethings you just can't *un-hear* either. Talk about UVI – unwanted visual image. I mentioned this encounter to the head nurse of the unit because I was concerned the resident had been taken advantage of, or possibly received a STI (sexually transmitted infection). The nurse spoke with the resident and assured me that they had been two consenting adults, and no harm was done.

Graduation into personal care homes brought me a whole new list of things to work on. There was a lot of M.S. (multiple sclerosis), Cerebral Palsy, Parkinson's, post-polio syndrome, hip and knee replacement surgeries, dementia, Alzheimer's and, of course, strokes and arthritis. I would treat my clients wherever they were most comfortable. Some were bedridden, or in a wheelchair, or Broda chair (a type of bed/chair), or even in a favorite recliner. We found a way to give them relief from their pain. I say "we" because massage therapy is a team effort between the client and the therapist.

Some couldn't speak but we found ways to communicate. Not all these people were elderly either. Some were my age and younger who had been in horrific accidents and lived to be completely dependent on caregivers. I learned to watch their breathing, how they held their bodies, their facial expressions, their eyes and even eyebrows for clues about what they were feeling.

College is a fantastic learning experience, but like a recipe book, it is just a place to start. Massage therapy as a profession is a learn-as-you-go procedure with instinct and common sense as your guide. One client in particular was a lady who was in a horrible accident. She had lost the use of her arms and legs, as well as part of her skull, all her teeth and bit off most of her tongue. Her ability to speak was extremely limited, but she had no trouble making it clear what she did or did not want! At first, she was in a lot of pain. Her neck was very swollen, and her head fell to one side from the missing muscles on the other side. Her ear had pressure sores on it from resting on her shoulder bone, and her neck muscles had shortened on that side, pulling her head down. It was going to be a challenge for sure.

Communication is a huge part of massage as well, but she couldn't speak so we had to find other ways… and we did. We began with reducing her swelling, which gave her comfort. Then we worked on opening the space between her ear and shoulder by relaxing and gently lengthening the neck muscles. Slowly, the space began to open. I started slipping rolled-up face cloths into the neck space to keep it open and help with perspiration. Then over time we graduated to a small pillow, and then a full pillow. I knew when it felt good to her because she would start to close her eyes. Then her breathing would slow down. Then her eyebrows would begin to lift higher and higher. Next came the involuntary muscle twitches in her arms and legs as she would start to fall asleep. And finally, her mouth would fall open. She taught me what true relaxation looks like and sounds like. These lessons were my most valuable lessons and I carry them with me to this day.

As a lucky result of treating folks in their beds at the personal care homes, I treated them as they were. My liability and malpractice insurance wouldn't allow me to position or turn my clients because I might get injured, and my insurance cancelled. The health care aids oversaw placing my clients in bed for their treatments. The majority of the time my clients were placed on their backs. Many of my clients complained about back pain so I had to be sneaky and slip my hand under the bottom sheet to get at their backs without turning them. A lot of the time I worked on shoulders and hips because they were laying face upward and I had noticed something. As I worked on their fronts, I happened to notice that their backs improved. This lucky happenstance would prove to be the basis for my future treatments.

They sat all day in their wheelchairs or recliners and their hips were getting tighter and tighter. They knitted or read or held their arms folded in front of them, all of which made their shoulders tighter and tighter. As these muscles were massaged, they became looser, and the shoulders became straighter. Their neck pain and upper backs didn't hurt so much anymore. As their hips and front leg muscles became looser and more relaxed, their back pain began to dissipate, and I hadn't even touched the back! I began to experiment with pillow placement and learned how to recline the wheelchairs back to let gravity help me with shoulder and hip massages. Clients had been slumping forwards as they relaxed in their wheelchairs and as a result their false teeth were falling out into their laps as they fell asleep.

Some wheelchairs have tables you can attach to them. Pillows on the table of a wheelchair would help the client sit back in their chair and support their shoulders. The recline, as well as the leg lifts, helped their knees and feet with swelling. All these features helped me massage. I would mimic this with pillows in their beds. Fortunately, most personal care beds are electric and have wonderful head and foot elevation capabilities. The beds could also go up and down making it easier for me to stand and not have to lean forward and hurt my back. As the bed would raise up from the ground, we would pretend we were on the escalator at the Bay downtown and going up to the different floors. We would start on the main floor, perfumes, scarves, hats and gloves. Second floor was men's furnishings. Next was china and crystal all the way up to the top floor. My clients would always giggle at the thought of riding the escalator, happy memories.

I realized the more they laughed at the beginning of the massage the faster they relaxed. Some people hold their breath when their muscles are sore. It's a natural reflex, but it makes the muscles stiffen. So, I would jokingly tell my seniors "whatever you do, don't stop breathing! I don't want you to relax *that* much." For some reason they found this morbid thought hilarious and, more often than not, they fell asleep. For some people it was the best sleep they got all week. The lights, the bells, the residents yelling or crying all night made it difficult to sleep. A precious 15 or 20 minutes during the massage were the deepest kind of sleep, and they really let it all go. Snoring, farting and drooling are all considered compliments to a massage therapist!

One of my most interesting experiences in personal care happened with a very strong-willed lady. She came across as very closed-off and kept to herself. One day she spoke to me and asked me to come massage her. She was in an electric wheelchair with a table attached. Her legs and feet were very swollen as were her arms and hands. Her head was also firmly attached to her right shoulder. Since I had seen this before, I knew what to do, or so I thought. This time was different. She had all her neck muscles, unlike my previous client who had this similar issue, but I could not find a reason for this drastic muscle imbalance. As she was most comfortable in her wheelchair for the massage treatments, we placed pillows onto her table to support her shoulders. I placed a towel over the pillows to protect them from getting lotion on them. We worked and worked on her neck twice a week with little progress. I was stumped! Over time, she opened up to me and began to share her stories of world travel with her beloved husband who had passed away ten years earlier. Although he was gone, you could tell she was still very much in love with him. Their adventures were fantastical, a true fairy tale.

One day we were getting set up for her treatment and she asked to have the radio on. She loved listening to oldies and classical music. We got her pillows and towel in place as we always did but something seemed different. She was softer, more vulnerable in a way. We began her massage, and the song "La Vie en Rose" came on the radio, I had heard all the wonderful stories of she and her husband's love of Paris. This song triggered something inside of her. This very controlled woman began to sob uncontrollably. Everything began to pour out of her. She apologized profusely as she grabbed tissue after tissue. I told her it was good to let it out and to not apologize. "Let it go," I coaxed. She poured and poured tears, and her body shook intensely. Then something amazing happened… her shoulder dropped! At the same time my mouth also dropped open. The injury in her shoulder she had been holding all this time was the pain from the loss of her husband. Ten years of not being able to grieve had manifested there.

As she finally allowed herself to grieve, I sat quietly holding her hand and supporting her. I had just witnessed a very private and personal moment of achievement and I felt so honoured that she shared that with me. This in medical terms is called a somatic release. And with somatic releases or emotional releases there can also be physical releases as well, and she proceeded to throw up… on herself and me. It went all the way down her front, across the pillow and up my chest and off the tip of my chin. Fortunately, I had closed my mouth by this time! She felt awful for making such a mess. I told her it was an incredible moment and got her cleaned up and changed her blouse. I too had to go home and get cleaned up and then back to work to continue my day. From that day forward massages with her were much easier. The shoulder and neck were no longer a problem. We continued our weekly massages until she joined her husband again.

Two other ladies, each with different types of brain injuries, were both affected on the right side of their bodies by paralysis. Their right arms were folded up into their shoulders with their joints flexed and curled inward. We call this a "spastic contracture." The brain injuries did not allow the nerves in their neck and spine to communicate with the muscles in their arms and legs properly. This type of treatment is slow and does not happen overnight. But they stuck with me, and we saw improvements with every massage, no matter how small. This wasn't a spa type of treatment either. There was some swearing involved… well from one of these ladies. My ears rang for a few days after the treatments with her. The other lady was far too sweet to swear, at least to my face. There was a lot of ice involved, or frozen peas to ease the pain. And they still stuck with me. It took years, with baby steps, but incredible things began to happen.

These ladies were about to teach me a new lesson but first I need to say these were only two cases where the nerves were not severed or dead. The pathways along their nerves were compromised by tight muscles and, as a result poor circulation. We were lucky to be able to override the nerves' impulses to contract constantly or not communicate properly. The spasms and swelling were reduced allowing the arm and hand to open, again, over time. This was a weekly or bi-weekly treatment to keep things moving in the right direction and not go back to the way it was.

Gradually the feeling began to come back, and the fingers began to move! With absolute and sheer stubbornness (some people call it determination, but let's call it what it is!), we soldiered on. Blood was flowing, muscles were relaxing, and exercises had begun. The nerves were getting the oxygen and nutrients they needed to heal. Nerves heal very slowly, which is a good thing. Have you ever frozen your foot in winter or slept on your hand and lost the feeling in it? Well, when it comes to, that is the feeling when nerves come back to life. Not pleasant, so it is better in small doses than all at once!

Arms were moving now and starting to take on new lives. The lady who swore at me was now phoning me! But instead of cursing me out she was speaking in a tone I'm pretty sure only dogs could hear.

"Slow down, slow down! I can't understand you" I'd say.

"I zipped up my own jacket!!" she yelled into the phone.

We cheered and celebrated over the phone for some time. It's amazing how much we take for granted. As much as I know I am stubborn, she was more so. I am certain that is the reason for her success. You get out what you put in, and she worked harder than anyone I had ever seen. She had an arm sling of sorts when we started to keep her shoulder from separating. That was gone now. Next, she started opening cans with an electric can opener. Just for fun try opening a can with an electric can opener with just one hand! Well now she had one and a half. Then it was washing her own clothes and changing her mattress cover on her bed, and cooking! Independence for a strong woman is heaven.

Then came the leg. We began working on the leg more once her arm and hand were improving. One day she told me her toes were tingling. During this time, she had gone from an electric wheelchair to a manual wheelchair as well as a cane and a brace on her leg. Independence was growing, and it was phenomenal to watch her progress. She was showering herself with home care present just in case. Eventually, she was walking just about everywhere with her cane, and the brace was only halfway up her calf now. The ankle had a hinge joint so she could bend her foot and use her muscles. She was getting stronger. Finally, she requested "No home care" and was granted it.

Meanwhile, my other lady was also continuing to improve. She was much older and had been living with the condition much longer. One Christmas to my surprise she presented me with knitted mittens and said, "We made these." Of course, I cried my eyes out. Each Christmas, the mittens got better and better and then came the fancy slippers with elaborate designs. But that first pair of mittens will always be my favorite.

She never did have a wheelchair and always used a walker with a leg brace. I attribute her success to her attitude. She had been through just about as much as any human can go through: the Second World War, relocating to another country, learning a new language, four children, loss of her spouse too early in life, her disability, and a few spinal fractures to top it all off. With all these reasons to give up or complain, she never did it once in the nineteen years I have been graced to work with her. Her favorite saying is "Do your best and leave the rest". So true.

One gentleman I worked with had been a teacher in the northern parts of Canada. He taught on the reserves in harsh climate. During the winter, he would stand on frozen concrete floors with nothing but a woodstove to heat the classroom. Over the years his feet suffered as the result of freezing and thawing on a daily basis. By the time he had retired, his feet were solid red bricks, and he was unable to walk. His feet were so red and swollen that not one joint in his ankles and feet would budge an inch.

Wheelchair ridden, his legs became stiff and stuck in a seated position as well. I was working close by, and his son contacted me to come work on his dad.

This poor man was in terrible shape. I began by massaging his hips and knees to open up the lines of circulation. His leg muscles were as hard as metal cables. Very slowly the blood flow began to increase. Movement in the hip and knee joints started. His poor hot swollen feet were finally able to start draining. It was slow but, bit by bit, his feet began to change colour from bright red to dark pink. Finally, the ankle joints started to budge, followed by the foot joints.

During our weekly treatments, I was entertained with stories of war time marches through the town of Brighton, England. He had been a soldier in the Second World War. My father had also grown up in Brighton, England and was obsessed with soldiers. At the time this gentleman was marching through the streets, my father would have been about twelve or thirteen years old and possibly saw him march by. As well, my client, who had moved to Canada after the war, had a love of all things RCMP. My father was sent over the ocean at the age of 15 to Canada and upon graduation from high school joined the RCMP. The parallel connections between these two men were fascinating to me. My client would talk about the Royal Canadian Mounted Police as a proud military type discipline. They would always salute with their right arm at their side with the longest way up and the shortest way down, meaning, the arm swung all the way up to their brow and cut short and quickly straight down the front of their face. He would always salute me at the end of our treatments that way as I was leaving, and I would salute him back.

After about three years this gentleman had improved so much that he was able to get out of his wheelchair. He graduated to a walker, and then a cane. One day he called me and was the most excited I had ever heard him. He told me that he had gotten to choose his own food at the lunch buffet. Normally, he had to wait for what he had chosen to be brought to him. That day he walked up to the table and chose for himself. He was thrilled.

The ten years I worked with "my seniors" in personal care homes were my most cherished and memorable years. There were a few bumps along the way though. All therapists at some point have to learn what their limits are. You cannot go from college to full-time work like most professions. You have to start slowly, build up your muscles, and become physically conditioned before you can work full time. Fortunately, most new therapists have to start slowly. As they build a clientele and as referrals begin to come in, it can sometimes be a painfully slow start, but it is better for the therapist.

Massage therapy is an extremely physical career, and you most undoubtedly will get injured if you don't take it slow. They say in college on day one, look to your left and look to your right: only one of you will finish this course. At the end of college, they again say, look to your left and look to your right: only one of you will make it past three years of practice. They are 100% right. Most massage therapists don't make it past year three of practice. They get injured, are unable to grow a clientele, or are disappointed with the money they make. You can't get into massage therapy thinking you will get rich!

Although it sounds like a huge amount per hour, you have expenses, and you can't work forty hours a week. Most therapists do between twenty to twenty-five hours per week, or less. If you try to work more, you will most likely get burnt out. That is what happened to me about year five after college. I was working five days a week with three personal care homes. My clientele was good, my business was booming, and I did not know where to draw the line. I was running on fumes doing over thirty hours of massage every week. My immune system was getting run down and working with people in such close proximity means you can easily catch a flu or cold. Somewhere along the way, whether I was hiking or just out enjoying the summer weather, I got bitten by a mosquito.

Getting bitten by a mosquito is a normal part of Canadian life, but this one had West Nile Virus in it. Some people get bitten by a mosquito with West Nile and only get flu-like symptoms if their immune system is strong. Some are hospitalized and even die from West Nile. I was very sick for nineteen months. Fortunately, I had good insurance and friends who helped me out with my work. One of my classmates from college had always wanted to get into personal care work, so I gave her one of my personal care homes, which helped me out greatly. For the other two personal care homes, I did what I could when I could. They were very understanding and supportive. A hard lesson learned: don't overdo it, listen to your body.

The last five years of my personal care home career went very well with my new understanding of what I could and could not do. During my tenth year in personal care, there was a terrible influenza outbreak in a lot of the personal care homes. I lost twelve clients in a month. This was too hard for me to handle. My heart was broken, and it was time for me to consider doing massage in another sector of the business. I decided to transition to clinical work. Over the next year, I eased my way out of personal care by not taking any new clients and working part-time at a spa. Finally, once I knew my personal care homes were set up with another therapist and my clients were left in good hands, and still keeping some of my clients in assisted living one day a week, I transitioned into clinical work.

CHAPTER TWO

Adventures of a Massage Therapist

As a massage therapist, a part of our certification and membership to an association requires us to continue our education. Which is great because personally I cannot learn enough about massage therapy. There are so many advances in massage therapy all the time that no one person will ever be able to learn it all in a lifetime. Conferences and study tours are two great ways to learn more about the different modalities and expand your knowledge base.

At one of my first massage therapy conferences there was a course on Quantum Somatics, which translates as "moving energy within the body." The premise is that humans, all matter, all have, and are made of energy, palpable and transferable energy. We all held hands in a circle, and the instructor held a light bulb of sorts that turned on when our hands were joined and off when we let go. I was a bit skeptical of course. Okay, I freely admit that I can be a bit of a "Doubting Debbie" when it comes to some treatment styles. Energy work was very foreign and a bit too "hocus pocus" to me in the beginning. Arms firmly crossed, with my head cocked to one side, and eyebrow lifted in disbelief, I thought: "Prove it to me."

The class lasted for three days during which the instructor talked about meridians, lights, wavy lines and colours we were supposed to be seeing. Meridians are lines in the body in which nerves, common pathways, and energy flow. Still doubting, but open to the possibility, I listened and learned. I had to admit I was starting to feel something. To me it felt like a warm and calming sensation. The words coming out of the instructor's mouth kept me skeptical, but the feelings kept me interested. I am the kind of person who needs hardcore proof. As the days passed and my arms unfolded it was undeniable: I felt it. I still couldn't see any wavy lines or lights, but I felt something moving and affecting the different areas of the body. This is the part where you or I would say, "It's all in your head!" Agreed, that went through my mind a hundred times.

When I got home to my practice and my seniors, I didn't tell them I was practicing energy work on them during the treatment. To my absolute surprise, the areas I was focusing and transferring the energy to relaxed! It was fast and without physical manipulation. This worked well on people who had a lot of swelling, an injury or recent surgery. The energy was relaxing their muscles where I wasn't able to apply pressure. Circulation increased, swelling went down, and limbs let go of tension, just with energy! My mind was officially blown.

I continue to this day to use this technique and some clients can feel it too without me telling them I am doing it. Most people cannot feel it or don't say anything if they do. There are people who are just more sensitive to it. I love it when a client asks me: "What did you just do there?!" I tell them it is energy work. They are surprised to hear that as they can feel the muscles releasing without me moving my hands. Listen, I don't expect you to understand this or even believe it, but it changed my mind and now I love to be proven wrong. That doesn't mean that I'm not a "Doubting Debbie" anymore, because I am. I just love to realize that if I knew that I knew nothing that would be something! There are things out there that we just don't or won't ever completely understand, but that doesn't mean they aren't real.

Over time, like any skill, you get better at it the more you practice it. There are times when I am massaging a client and their endorphins are flowing, and they start to feel like they are floating. It's a place between awake and falling asleep. As I share the energy with them, I sometimes begin to see colours, not like an aura on the outside of the body… personally, I am not able to see that… yet… and maybe never will. Nor have I ever seen the lines they talked about in the course. It is like an internal display of beautiful blues, pinks and purples when I close my eyes. At times I can catch a ride and feel the floating sensation from my client. Those who study chakras (energy centres in the body) say that the blues, pinks and purples are connected to consciousness and extrasensory perception. There is no religion in this at all. It is very simply the energy we all have in our bodies.

In 2016, ten years after the Quantum Somatics course, I travelled to Hawaii to study Lomi Lomi, which means to knead, rub or massage with aloha in Hawaiian. Hawaii has always been a magical place for me. My father and his second wife lived there for seventeen years on their protea flower farm on Kilauea Mountain. I hadn't been back to the Big Island since my father passed in 2000 but I was able to find his farm with the house he and his wife built. It was amazing to me because there had been a horrible vog (volcanic fog) five or six years earlier that had been blown up the side of the mountain and killed most of the protea flower farms. I was worried that my father's labour of love had been erased. To my delight, it was one of the few that had survived, and it was blooming!

I was sixteen years old the first time I visited my father and had taken photos of the island and mainly the town of Kilua, Kona. It was now 2016, thirty-two years later and I had the idea of finding all the places I had taken pictures of on my first visit and making a before-and-after photo album. I had a few days to myself before the course began so, with a clipboard and photos in plastic sleeves, I began to search out the original spots. It wasn't easy because things change a lot in thirty-two years. Every morning, I woke early excited to explore the town again. I would get myself a Kona coffee and start to search out the familiar places I had so many beautiful memories of. In Hawaii no one starts work until 10 a.m. It was just me and the street sweepers up that early.

As I wandered through the town and snapped my photos, I noticed that one of the shops in the village was just opening its doors. It was 9:45 a.m. and none of the other shops were open yet. This was a ukulele store, and a young woman came to the door and asked me if I would like to come in. I gladly accepted and popped into the store. She said that she never got there that early. I thought it was such a coincidence that I had been walking by just as she was opening her store. I looked around and couldn't find anything because it was too expensive for me. As I browsed through her store, she said to me "I see you have some photos there, may I see them?" Gladly I showed them to her. As she flipped through the pictures she stopped and pointed at one of them.

"I know this man!" she said.

I looked at her and told her there was no way she could have known him. That picture was from 1984, it had been 32 years since it was taken and there was no way she was that old. She smiled at me and told me she was 40 years old. To me she looked mid-twenties to thirty at the most.

"This was my parents shop when I was a little girl. And your father and his wife were always just over there," she said, pointing in the direction of a shop Dad's wife worked at. She told me how she would go visit them all the time. I asked her what her name was. "Rosebud" she replied. I couldn't believe it, my father with his signature giggle, would tell us delightful stories about this sweet little girl named Rosebud who would hang out with them. Dad was friends with everyone who he crossed paths with, but this little girl had made an impression on him and his wife enough to tell us about her.

She and I talked for quite a while and not only did she run the ukulele shop, sing and write music, but as it turned out she was a massage therapist too! She practiced Lomi Lomi massage there as well and that is why I had come. What an incredible coincidence! We exchanged info and parted ways with a hug.

Next was Dad's tennis club. This is where his memorial had been held. Several people came to it. Again, I spoke to no one and just looked around, imaging my father playing tennis there. A woman approached me, and I thought she was going to tell me to leave because it was a private club.

But instead, she said, "I see you have some photos there; may I see them?"

I thought, "Okay, this is getting weird." But I shared the pictures with her and, low and behold, she recognized my father.

"I know this man, he used to play here."

Others joined in, and the heart-warming stories began to flow. It was wonderful to me that so many people remembered him so fondly after 16 years! Again, the lady and I exchanged info and said good-bye with a hug.

Next stop was the condo my father used to manage as one of his first jobs in Hawaii. I spent some time there and had a flood of good memories. There was a lady doing maintenance of the grounds and trimming hedges and she kept watching me. Probably thinking I was up to no good...or so I thought. She made her way over to me and you will never guess what she said!

"I see you have some photos there; may I see them?"

Now, not that that wasn't the theme of the day, but I thought who says that as an opening to a conversation? I stopped second-guessing what was happening and gladly showed her the pictures. As it turned out she had been the caretaker there for over 35 years. She introduced herself and the name rang a bell for me. I recalled her being there when I was 16. She began to name all my siblings and remembered me too. We talked for some time and I took her photo at the condo entrance way and we said good-bye with a hug.

Some of my father's ashes were placed at a spot in Hawaii called South Point. I went there a few times with him and others. It was one of his favorite places to go. I had the idea to buy some protea flowers, the kind he grew, and place them at South Point as a bit of a memorial of my own. Due to the vog incident, there were none to be found for sale. I was extremely disappointed.

On my way out to South Point, I stopped at a town called Ocean View that was the closest town to the farm. Again, I found no protea, nor did I have any ideas about where I could find some. I wandered across the parking lot to a gift shop and thought maybe I could find some gifts for friends back home there. A woman, obviously not in a good mood, was working behind the counter there. She asked me gruffly, "what are you looking for?"

I told her I didn't know and would just look around, although my instinct was to just leave. I found some cute cards and was really enjoying reading them. They were hilarious to me and I found myself laughing out loud. Then I noticed some beautiful, handcrafted wind chimes that were exactly what one of my clients asked me to bring back for her, but they were too high for me to reach. I had to ask the surly lady to help me. Still not happy she helped me begrudgingly. I asked her as she was retrieving the wind chime I had selected if she knew where I could find some protea flowers to buy.

She, in true form, replied, "There are none."

"How about other flowers?" I asked.

"We have none", she snapped.

As I walked up to the counter to pay for the cards and the wind chime, I placed the clipboard with the photos on the counter. I caught her glancing at them out of the corner of her eye as she rang up my purchases. Her son had just shown up with her lunch, well after 1 p.m. and her attitude became clear to me…she was hangry. She kept looking at the pictures and finally she said it…

"I see you have some photos there; may I see them?" I was surprised to hear this, especially from her. As she looked through the pictures she said "I know these people! They lived right up the mountain there," she said as she pointed to the direction of my father's farm.

I explained that the man in the photo was my father, and that I wanted to put flowers out on South Point where some of his ashes are. She took me by the hand and led me out to another room just off to the side of the shop. There were potted

Bougainvillea bushes there. She told me to pick one. I was thrilled and excited to finally have the vibrant pink, delicate flowers. They were perfect. I thanked her and although we forewent the hug, I could see in her eyes she had softened. I continued on my way and, after placing the flowers lovingly in a perfect nook in the lava and having a little private conversation with Dad, I continued my journey to the Kalani retreat for my Lomi Lomi training.

The directions I was given to the retreat were not the best, so finding the retreat was possibly one of the most nerve racking, leap of faith moments of my life. They told me, "Drive until you pass the two trees on the left after the building that used to be a church."

I hoped I had picked the right road, because there were many trees and buildings that could have been the ones they were talking about, and of course the roads don't have names. Now I am driving down this seemingly endless dirt road with the ocean on one side and random illegible signs on the other. There is no such thing as a straight flat road in Hawaii either, so I am driving up hills and around sharp corners next to this cliff down to the ocean while trying to read these weather-beaten signs. Locals drive really fast on these roads, so I am watching out for them too and trying not to veer into on-coming traffic.

The trip took longer than I had thought, and I began to worry that I was on the wrong road and would have to turn around and go all the way back to start over. I saw a small spot to pull off the narrow two-lane road and ask for directions. Two kind people were strolling along, and I asked them if they knew where Kalani retreat was. They looked at me with a stunned look on their faces. They pointed across the road to a small orange flag. "It's right there, Miss," the kind people said. With much embarrassment I thanked them and turned into the driveway of the Kalani retreat.

After registering at the retreat office and getting the key to my bungalow, I unpacked and made my way to the Rainbow Room for orientation. This was a huge quonset-type building with screened walls at each end to let the Hawaiian breeze blow through. It was made of some kind of wood and was incredibly peaceful and calming. You could hear the waves crashing on the cliffs across the road like a constant white noise that was soothing. And, as always in Hawaii, there was the fragrance of saltwater and flowers that enchanted every moment.

To my surprise there were twenty-eight other participants besides myself. They were from all over the world; only two of us were Canadian. Some spoke little to no English, but massage is a universal language in and of itself. Not everyone was a massage therapist either. There were yogis, doctors, and the curious. None of us had any idea what Lomi Lomi was truly about, but we all felt a "need" to be there. The need to go for some was so powerful that they had quit their jobs because they couldn't get the time off. The stories began. Everyone had a painful story of deep-seated wounds from losses, rejection, and/or breaking free of controlling situations. We were all there to heal ourselves and each other. Over the next eight days, each and every one of us shared, supported and healed together. After each training session we would sit together in a circle and share our experiences that we'd had during the session. There were tears, gentle kindnesses, and acceptance within our circle every day.

It was a safe place to learn and heal together. Our instructors were well trained in helping us sort out and understand where these feelings were coming from and how to love ourselves as we released the pain and emotions. One instructor described "people" as bowls of light when we are born. As we learn and grow, people we know and love put rocks in our bowls by telling us we can't do something, or we'll never be able to do something. Negative judgements are rocks blocking out our light. Lomi Lomi was teaching us how to take these rocks out of our bowls to let the light shine through again. Forgiving others, ourselves and loving ourselves was our mantra.

The Hawaiian people believe that they live in two realms, the earthly and the spiritual. They also believe that through Lomi Lomi we can tap into our spiritual realm and visit our past and future selves for guidance and the giving of support. Lomi Lomi massage is not religion based, but assistance to help the recipient open up the areas of their body that hold their deep-seated pain and release it. It's called "weeding your emotional garden." Emotional pain or "rocks" in our bowl can manifest into physical pain and create imbalances in the body. The lady who lost her husband and was unable to grieve is a classic example of how pain can create a physical manifestation.

In Lomi Lomi, there are two practitioners, one working on each side of the recipient at the same time. This overloads the recipient's brain with stimulation and allows it to open up to receive "Aloha" or loving support from your future and past selves as well as your ancestors. Once the mind is open to assistance the weeding begins. The practitioners begin to open up the chakras, or energy centres, through a type of flushing motion.

This type of massage therapy is hundreds of years old, and we had to receive permission from the local Kahuna or Hawaiian chief to learn and carry forward their sacred practices. Hawaiians believe that we become connected to our spiritual selves by pressing into the bones. As we did this, some of my classmates were reporting having visions! Of course, the "Doubting Debbie" in me reappeared. Some were exploring the universe, and others were going back to the womb in their "visions." Sure, whatever, I thought.

It was around day six when we were practicing the facial component of the Lomi Lomi. A classmate, with whom I had become good friends, was my partner. She and her husband were from somewhere near Russia. They were lovely people with gentle kind spirits. He practiced massage therapy, and she was a massage therapist, general practitioner, an herbalist, as well as a psychiatrist back home. They spoke little English, but we communicated just fine. The facial massage in Lomi Lomi is a ten-minute treatment near the end of the massage.

As my classmate began to work on me, gently pressing into my cheek bones and eye socket bones, it happened! I zipped out of my body and plain as day saw a vision. It was only a second or two but there was zero doubt about what had just happened to me. I opened my eyes and looked at my classmate and said, "I'm pretty sure I just had my first vision!" It was not as profound as some the others had, but I saw this beautiful field of golden wheat with the bluest sky and dirt road. There were five stainless steel metal mailboxes with the red flags up. Honestly, I was in shock at first. It was too fast to be a dream and it was so vivid. I felt myself lift out of my body. I felt stunned and confused. What did it mean? I finally had a vision. Others had gone flying through the universe and back to their mother's womb, and I got five mailboxes in a field! Probably in Saskatchewan! Really! That's it!

People laughed at my story and my exasperation. The instructors tried not to giggle and reassured me that its meaning would become clear to me eventually if I just sat with it. Umm, okay... so far, nothing.

Lomi Lomi is practiced on a bare vinyl table. The reason for the bare table is so that the practitioners can slide their hands under your back. The massage is done almost completely with the soft part of the forearm just below the elbow. Lotion is used to glide the forearms up and down the length of the body. The hands are only used when sliding up and down the spine while the recipient is lying on his or her back, and for the facial portion. The only sheet is the one that covers you at the end of the treatment.

The chakras are down the centre of the body from the top of your head to the bottom of your torso. Access to the chakra areas is important in order to help open them up. When performing Lomi Lomi the recipients, male and female, are normally bare chested. A consent form is signed by the women to allow the treatment. At no time is the breast area massaged, but the area between the breasts is the heart chakra, and it is less effective to have a towel or sheet there. There is a small diaper-type covering for the genitals and bum areas as well.

In order to prepare for this portion of the class, we all went to a clothing optional black sand beach nearby. Some people had no problem with the nudity. Being a lily-white Canadian, my only concern was burning my parts, the ones that had rarely ever seen the sun. There was another Canadian gal there, and we sat in our one-piece bathing suits with hats and towels wrapped around us while slathering on suntan lotion. It was February, and our delicate Canadian skin would have blistered in no time flat. At least I had a partner in this because most others ran around with breasts and penises flying everywhere. I have no problem with nudity; I'm just opposed to sunburns. If you have ever received a massage with a sunburn, you'll understand. Actually, the only problem I had was when people came right up to us sitting on the beach. They were naked and standing much too close. As you can imagine, certain parts were eye level to us, and it made it exceedingly difficult to maintain eye contact.

The retreat itself was a large, gated community run completely by volunteers. All the buildings, gardens, animals and meals were tended to and prepared by the hands of the volunteers who, in exchange, lived room and board free. Everything came from the land. There were fruit trees, garden vegetables, and freshly caught seafood daily. The animals and dairy were processed within 25 miles of the retreat. There were four chefs who prepared our three meals a day, one of whom had previously worked for the Queen of England.

Our meals were announced by three blows of a conch shell. The meals were large buffet style and offered something for everyone. There were salads with homemade dressing, fruit juices blended from the fruit trees on the property, and desserts made from the roasted cocoa beans and macadamia nuts on the grounds. It was heaven! Besides the amazing meals the grounds offered a pool and hot tub.

It was a dry retreat, so no drugs or alcohol were allowed. There was a designated spot for cigarette smokers and no cell service. There were land line phones if you needed to make a call. The idea was to be mindful in the moment and be in tune with nature. There were semi-wild pigs and piglets running around as well as tame cats to keep the mouse population down. Adorable little green and blue geckos were also everywhere keeping the cockroaches to a minimum. Colourful tropical birds lived in the jungle that came right up to the property. At night, the streams that flowed from the jungle were full of frogs that sang me to sleep.

After a day of massaging and eating in the endless humidity, all I had the power to do was shower and go to bed. The jetlag woke me up daily at 4 a.m. It was my favorite part of the day. I would get my coffee and a guava juice and stroll down to the hot tub. No one but the morning staff preparing breakfast was up. There were very few lights, so we had little flashlights on our key chains. The grounds were safe, and the trails were magical in the dark. I would go sit in the hot tub in the dark morning moonlight completely alone. The full moon laid flat on its side down there as its light shone through the palm trees. It was so beautiful I felt like I was in a movie or a painting. The stars were very bright as well. Orion was enormous in the night sky! I could see the stars so clearly in the darkness of the retreat. I found new constellations like the brachiosaurus and one that looked like a full crab made up of hundreds of stars, and all the while the waves crashing in the distance…magical.

After eight amazing days it was finally time to say good-bye. With hugs and tears, we finished our course, each back to our own realities again, but better prepared to face it. Our busy lives took over again, but the memories of our Hawaiian adventure continue to visit me regularly.

Two years later, Thailand was the next adventure. My massage therapy association put together a study tour. Twelve massage therapists from across Canada signed up, and we began our journey west. We all met in Vancouver, B.C. and were supposed to all get on a China Airlines flight together; however, my name and one other massage therapist's name were not on the confirmation list. The other massage therapist was able to purchase the last seat on the flight. I was not so lucky. As I watched my class-mates board the plane, I began to worry that I would never get there. They waved good-bye and wished me luck. I needed some, but it was almost midnight on a Friday, and my association's office was closed, and they were in the process of moving to a new building that weekend as well. The travel agency was also closed so there was no one I could get ahold of. The lovely people at the China Airlines desk helped me to arrange a hotel room nearby the airport for the night.

I got to my hotel room starving and emotionally exhausted. I started texting and emailing everyone in the association office for whom I had contact information. There was an emergency phone number set up for the transition weekend and, thankfully, I had written it down! I called and left several messages, as I kept running out of time on the answering machine. At 2:00 or 3:00 a.m., I took a shower and laid down to rest.

The hotel was not the nicest one I had ever been in, that's for sure. I could hear everything through the walls. There was a man in the next room with three young prostitutes! He kept asking one of them her age. She said it was fine, that she was old enough, but he decided to make her leave. She pounded on his door for at least 10 minutes. He finally told her she had to go. Then the three of them proceeded with the night's activities. Fortunately, I had packed ear plugs. A few hours later I was awoken by multiple text messages and emails! The association had received my messages and were already on it! I spoke with the association and the travel agent several times that morning getting things straightened out. After a nice breakfast at the hotel, I cabbed back to the airport for an 11:00 a.m. flight to Thailand. They were amazing and apologized so many times for the mistake.

I ended up getting booked with a more expensive airline and was treated very well. The flight was from Vancouver to Korea, a quick plane change, and then straight on to Chiang Mai where my classmates were. I dined on shrimp salad, steak, potatoes and complimentary wine. The flight was uneventful, which is a good thing; however, the head wind was extraordinarily strong. We were going to be late into Korea.

The stewardess let me know that I was going to miss my connecting flight to Chiang Mai. I became really worried. I couldn't speak Korean, and the Winter Olympics were being hosted in Seoul, where we were landing. There was no way I would get a hotel room this time. I dreaded the thought of having to go through all of that again. The calling, the texting, the emails, and the waiting… Uggh! Feeling very sorry for myself, I disembarked the plane and dragged my sad bum through the airport thinking I'd have to sleep there. Then I saw a lady holding a sign. It had my flight number and Chiang

Mai written on it. I quickly checked my ticket to make sure I wasn't hallucinating. I felt like I had just won the lottery! I went up to her and showed her my ticket, and she rushed me through the airport to my gate. They apologized for the fact that the flight was late in leaving, but I laughed: I couldn't believe my good luck. Within 15 minutes, I was on my way to Chiang Mai! I texted our contact in Thailand just before we left, and he said he would meet me at the airport. As it turned out I arrived two hours after my classmates who left before me! The next morning, I surprised my classmates, who were unaware that I had made it in, and joined them for breakfast. It turned out their flight had not been that great. They'd had sandwiches for dinner and an eight-hour layover in the Bangkok airport.

After breakfast we had a free day to get to know one another and tour around Chiang Mai. The annual flower festival was on that weekend, so we had a real treat to welcome us. Our fearless leader, who had been there before, walked us all over the city. We went to one of his favorite restaurants. It had decorative walls and clay pots scattered about a tropical outdoor dining area. It was like a scene from *Indiana Jones* or *Laura Croft Tomb Raider*. The food was amazing too. We continued our walking tour to the flower festival grounds.

After an hour or so, we regrouped to head over to the city's market. There were people everywhere! Shoulder to shoulder, we clumped together and bumped our way through the enormous market until our jetlag started to kick in, and we headed back to our lovely hotel. Someone had kept track of our steps on her phone that day; we walked over 26,000 steps! We were tired.

On day one of eight school days, we met downstairs in our hotel lobby after break-fast and proceeded to climb into the back of a truck. It had a topper on it with two benches and a metal rail to hold on to. All twelve of us squished in together, the tailgate was closed, and off we went to our first day of Thai massage training. It was about half an hour drive to and from school each day. For the first three days we just screamed as the cars, mopeds, and trucks were driving all over the place. There didn't seem to be any order at all, and we were certain we were going to die in a fiery crash. They zipped in and out of lanes — no helmets, sometimes babies, pets and groceries on board — with up to five people per moped! Being their winter in Thailand, the same time as ours, they were wearing toques and down filled jackets. It was 32 degrees Celsius, and we were melting! After about three days, we got used to the chaos of the local drivers and stopped screaming. We realized that there was method to their madness; we never once saw an accident.

Our Thai massage classes were steeped in tradition, with techniques passed down over hundreds of years from the monks. We washed our feet at the beginning of each session. Then we joined in the chanting of prayers in Thai each morning before classes began. We were given special clothes to wear each day, and they laundered them for us each night. Lunch was an adventure in itself. The massage school was across the highway from a marketplace. You had to cross 10 lanes of traffic successfully if you wanted food. It was terrifying the first couple of times because not everyone stops for you. In fact, there was an entire class on our first day devoted to how to cross the road. You have to stick your arm out. If the first lane stops, you have to step out in front of them and stick out your arm and wait for the next lane to stop and so on until you get across all five lanes and onto the median. Then you have to do it all over again for the traffic coming from the opposite direction. To make things more confusing, people drive on the right side of the car, and traffic flows in the opposite directions from Canada. This too became old hat and easy after a few days.

Considering how aggressive they are with their driving, Thai people are the kindest, most respectful people I have ever met. I can't speak for Bangkok, but in Chiang Mai up north near the foothills of the Himalayas, with all the farmland and temples, the people are so kind. If you bump into a Thai person, which happens a lot there, they will apologize to you with hands together and a bow. Hordes of people bumping into each other and bowing and apologizing everywhere! After a short period of time, we were doing this too. Besides the sweet, endearing people, the food was my favorite thing. For 50 baut, which was then about $2 Canadian, you could have a huge meal. Everything is brought in fresh daily from the farms. Spices, herbs, greens, and fruits are all picked ripe and sold that day. Fresh bananas and coconuts were also everywhere. As a class we toured the countryside and visited temples, an elephant sanctuary, and nature parks.

Most Thai people have at least two or three jobs. They work extremely hard for little pay. Some work as many as 20 hours per day! They don't sit at desks all day like a lot of Canadians. They are small people with hard lives. Many will pick rice in a field all day. Thai massage is tailored to small people with hard muscles. I think it is fair to say that dehydration is also a problem for Thai people. They live in a hot, humid country in which they work hard, and clean drinking water is scarce.

As Canadians, we outweigh most of them by 50 to 100 pounds. We live very luxurious lives compared to the Thai.

I think it is also fair to say that most Canadians cannot bend as well as Thai people. They put you on a mat on the floor and place you in yoga-type positions and then begin to massage you. They will use their knees, elbows and feet with their full weight on you. Personally, I would break my clients if I used my full body weight on them.

We worked incredibly hard for eight days in rooms with little to no air conditioning as it was their winter, and they were wearing sweaters. A constant stream of sweat poured down our backs. The only relief we had was the freezing cold pool back at our hotel that we raced to at the end of each day. By the end of our classes most of us were black and blue and felt like hamburger.

Thailand was a completely different world from Canada, and I encourage people to visit there, but one bit of advice: the washrooms in public areas are an adventure in and of themselves! If you are lucky, you get an actual toilet seat and even luckier if there is toilet paper. Some public washrooms consist of a trough with channels carved into the floor. You just have to hope your aim is good and you don't get any on your shoes. Other times there are faux bidets made up of a hose and spray nozzle. Sometimes you have to pay for the pleasure of this experience. So, my advice to you is… bring wet wipes and hand sanitizer.

Not every course is something you take forward into your practice. Sometimes learning what you don't want to do is just as important and valuable. For some of my classmates, Thai massage was just the thing they were searching for. Although I do not practice Thai massage, the experience of learning about another culture's traditions and healing techniques was an opportunity of a lifetime. Because of their generosity and peaceful ways, no one goes hungry in a country of 68 million people. Everyone shares and shows respect. That is what I will carry forward with me.

CHAPTER THREE

Breathe and Relax

D on't let anyone tell you that relaxing is easy.

We come out of our mothers kicking and screaming and then try to figure out how to relax every day after that. Everyone has the ability to do it. It just takes an enormous amount of concentration. After enough practice you can get good at anything, even relaxing. The real challenge comes when someone, hopefully a thera pist of some sort, is digging into your hip or armpit.

The first key to relaxing is breathing. When we are in pain our first instinct is to hold our breath. Some people are shallow breathers and only take air into part of their lungs. When you breathe you should fill up your lungs completely. The lower lobes of your lungs are all the way down near your stomach. When you fill your lungs, it should feel like your stomach is filling up with air. Lying down on your back and taking a full breath should make your stomach rise. The speed of your breath is important too. Whether you choose to breathe through your nose or mouth, it should take 3-4 full seconds to inhale and 3-4 seconds to exhale. There should be no stopping or holding of breath in between the inhale and the exhale. The air should come in and go out in a continuous, slow moving action. This action keeps the ribs moving as we breathe. That is important because so many muscles attach to the ribs. When we stop the air or hold our breath, our muscles naturally stiffen.

Breathing also provides our muscles with the oxygen they need to relax. If you breathe too fast you will get dizzy and lightheaded. Fast breathing and holding your breath do not help the therapist during a massage, especially a "therapeutic" massage. It actually slows down the treatment. Relaxing tight muscles can be painful at times and communication with your therapist is crucial to insure you are both on the same page. A therapist can tell when you are tight, or when an area is swollen or painful by the feel and temperature of the tissues. Typically, we try to get the tight muscles into a slight stretch in order to activate the receptors in the tendons.

Your therapist can tell if a muscle is at its maximum stretch point or "end point." Normally, we feel the resistance in the muscle we are stretching and estimate the level of pain or discomfort you are feeling. On a scale of 1-10, 1 being no pain and 10 being the most awful thing you've ever experienced, we aim for about a 7. A "7" is just before "too much": tolerable, but not comfortable. I like to say to my clients that it's like I am taking them to the edge of the cliff but not pushing them over.

It's at this point that communication is crucial. When you are at the "7" point of a therapeutic massage, if at any point it starts to go past the 7 and starts climbing to an 8, 9 or 10, you must let your therapist know. We can normally tell when this is happening by the way people hold their bodies like, for example, clenching their teeth, arching their lower backs, pressing their heads backward onto the table and holding their breath. People have different tolerance levels. They may be more sensitive or less sensitive. What feels like a 5 or 6 to a therapist may feel like a 7 or 8 to the client, or vice versa. What feels like a 7 or 8 to the therapist may only feel like a 5 or 6 to the client. That is when communication is especially important. So, the big question – the most common one I get is: how do you relax?

This explanation will help. Relaxing is the absence of tension or stimulation to the muscle. None of your muscles should be flexing or "holding". Being aware that you are holding your muscles is half the battle. When you are relaxed, your body should fall or flop. Gravity is in control of you now. When your head is resting and relaxed it is heavy. Like resting on a pillow: zero effort. Your head will naturally fall to one side or the other.

Your neck, however, is the *most* difficult part of your body to relax because it is so very mobile and also very vulnerable. There are so many nerves and major blood vessels and arteries there that our natural instinct is to protect the neck all the time.

Because so many people hold their stress in their necks, it is often a difficult job for therapists to gain the trust we need to effectively release and relax the neck muscles. This is why I save it until the last part of the treatment with some clients. Once the rest of your body is loose and relaxed it is much easier to relax your neck. Clients who are familiar with their therapist's treatment style are more likely to trust them with their necks and have to ability to let them go. It is exceedingly difficult to override muscle instincts, which is why I say massage therapy is a team effort. Sometimes it takes everything you've got, and everything I've got combined, to help a muscle release, especially if it is painful or in spasm.

A spasm is a muscle that has been stretched too far and so the body's response to that is to pull the muscle back to where it should be comfortably. The brain and spinal cord keep sending out messages along the nerves of the over stretched muscle to contract. It is like holding down the "e" key on your keypad, eeeeeeeeee. For each "e" on the pressed keyboard, the nerve sends out a contraction message to the muscle. A spasm is the body's way of trying to protect the muscle from being torn and damaged. It is incredibly difficult to release a spasm and having these relaxing skills will help the therapist attempting to release it.

Trying to let go of control in your arms and legs is also very hard to do. We use them constantly for everything. Our arms and hands move all the time without us being aware of it. They balance us as we sit and walk. Some people talk with their hands and mouth at the same time. Trying to control this takes a lot of concentration. I used to joke with my seniors who used their hands while they talked. I told them I would have to find a big heavy book to put on their hands to keep them still. Finally, a use for their encyclopedias! Again, they laughed at my stupid joke, and it helped them remember to keep their hands still.

When hands and fingers move it effects the muscles all the way up to your neck. Back muscles have to become rigid to stabilize the body so that the arms can move. Otherwise, we would be flopping all over the place when we moved our arms. When we move our arms around while standing, the neck and back muscles all become rigid to stabilize the body and keep the eyes still so we can focus. When the back is rigid the legs, are affected and become tighter. And so on, and so on. Everything is truly connected. So, when I ask a client to stop moving their fingers during a neck or leg massage, they are always surprised that I can tell. "Busted!"

When an arm is relaxed, it should fall as if it were dead weight. Of course, we won't let it fall, that's where trust comes in again. Letting it all go is hard. The trick is knowing which muscles are holding the limb tight or protecting it. It is our job as therapists to let you know where you need to focus your relaxation. Many times, if a hand or elbow are having trouble relaxing, my clients will try to shake it out of their arm or hand but that never helps anything relax. Getting the client to relax their shoulder often helps relax the elbow and hand muscles.

Leg muscles are the largest muscles in the body. They can be incredibly strong. The best way to relax leg muscles is also the "let gravity have its way" approach. If I need to push on the outside of the leg, rolling it towards the other leg, it should roll back on its own without any assistance. That is true relaxation. If I lift the leg up off the table, the foot should drop with gravity. If not, the thigh muscles are contracted and keep the knee straight, and this is not relaxation. If I lift the arm up to move it and it stays up in the air without me holding it, this is not relaxation. After a few massages you become more aware of your body and the tightness in it. You are able to know which muscles are working unnecessarily and let them go. You conserve a lot of energy when you are able to let them go consciously and, therefore, have more energy for the rest of your day.

Some other great ways to become more aware of your body are yoga and mindfulness. Yoga helps you breathe and feel the places that are tight. Yoga stretches and strengthens every muscle in your body. Most athletes use some type of yoga stretches to warm up before their game. Mindfulness is being aware of what is happening in the moment: how you are breathing, feeling, what you are hearing or smelling. Meditation and mindfulness apps with music can help you focus on your breath and different areas of the body and consciously relax them.

Getting enough water for your muscles is crucial too. Coffee, teas and juices are diuretics. They make you pee more than you are taking in. For each cup (250 ml) of coffee you drink, you pee more than a cup, so you are becoming dehydrated. For each cup of coffee, tea or juice, you need to have a cup of water to replace the eliminated water, and then you need to consume your daily intake of water on top of that. Everyone is different with water requirements. When you work out, do a physical job, sweat, breathe, pee or go #2, you lose water. If your pee is dark yellow, or you have to keep clearing your throat by "um-humming", that means you need to drink more water.

When we breathe, we bring in oxygen and breathe out CO_2 (carbon dioxide), which is waste or a toxin. When we void or evacuate our bowels that is waste and toxins too. When we drink enough water in a day it helps our bodies flush out these toxins. If someone is constipated their body is holding on to too much toxin. We can become lethargic and moody when we have too much toxin in our bodies. Muscles, especially leg muscles, can hold a lot of toxins in them because they are the largest muscles, and it is more work for the body to pump the blood up through them into the body to be processed. Blood can become stagnant, and toxins build up in the legs very easily. This is why stretching is so important after a big workout or run. It helps to flush the blood that builds up in the legs out and therefore the toxins.

By the way, your nose is another great way to tell when you have too much toxin in your body. If you get a stuffy nose during a massage, it is your body's reaction to the toxin, one which produces histamines. We take antihistamines for allergies. This histamine reaction is your body's way of asking you to drink more water and flush it out. When you get a massage, it is important to be hydrated before the treatment in order to effectively flush these toxins out of your body. Otherwise, you can get a "stuffy" nose or head. You should also drink enough water after a massage as well as the day after, to rehydrate which will make your pee a light yellow or almost clear. Massage therapists can also let you know when you are dehydrated by the hardness of your muscles, the look of your skin and if their hearing is really good, the sounds your eyes and mouth make. They sound clicky when they are too dry.

CHAPTER FOUR

The Body Mechanic

Over the last eighteen years, twenty if you include college, and forty-eight if you count all the years before college, I began to see patterns when I was treating a client. As humans we are pretty predictable. We work, we play sports, exercise, sleep, and raise our children. All of these activities have patterns. For example, if you work at a desk all day, you sit most of the day and as humans we cannot sit properly all day without get tired. We slouch or lean to one side or the other. Muscles lengthen and shorten as we use them or misuse them over long periods of time. It's a part of our evolutionary process. If you repeat a pattern for a long period of time, like sitting, our hip muscles where we bend will begin to shorten. The muscles and tendons get bunched up like a bendy straw. Over time our body starts to make these muscles shorter to keep us comfortable.

There are little spider web-type connective tissues in our bodies called "adhesions." They form and grow in between our muscles to help solidify these prolonged positions. Our bodies are constantly building up the areas of repetitive use or misuse to make us happy and comfortable, or so it thinks. If you have ever had a cast on a broken limb you will know what I mean. Let's say you broke your arm, and the cast keeps your elbow in a bent position. The body makes the elbow "happy" by shortening the muscles and tendons and solidifying the joint with adhesions. When the cast comes off it is difficult to straighten the elbow. It is the same for any joint you repetitively bend for long periods of time. Not only do we sit for work, but in our cars, watching TV, working on our home computers, eating, or even sleeping curled up. Our hips only bend one way comfortably, forward. If you add up all the time, we have our hips bent into an L shape in a day and possibly at night, it is a lot. And if you add up all of the years you have done this repetitive action, you can see how these adhesions build up. As our hip muscles get shorter and shorter over time, this causes our body to lean forward when we stand up. Some people, especially the elderly, lean forward a lot when they walk. They have had many more years of sitting and adhesions building up, so much so, you can actually see the lean. This is what is happening to the majority of us unless we are stretching these tight hip muscles daily. Adhesions form every day; therefore, we have to stretch and keep them broken up every day. Otherwise, they will build up to a point where joints become less mobile and create imbalances in our bodies. We are machines in a way that need to keep moving, or we will seize up. Have you ever heard the saying, "if you rest, you rust?" Well, it couldn't be any truer.

One of the hardest concepts I have had to try to get across to my clients over the years is the fact that we only bend one way, forwards. We don't bend backwards easily, well unless you are a gymnast or with Cirque du Soleil. We drive, we sit to type and text, we sleep, cook, hold our babies and hug our loved ones. Everything is bending forward. Our hips and shoulders all pull inwards towards our centres. Even our necks are getting into the action more lately looking down at our smart phones. We are slowly imploding forward tighter and tighter. In a tug of war between our front muscles and back muscles, the front will win every time because we use them constantly. It makes sense, right?

So why do our backs hurt if the front muscles are the tight ones? Good question! There are two kinds of tight muscles. There are the shortened muscles that more or less resemble knots for the purpose of visual explanation. When you tie knots in a rope it gets shorter. The other kind of tight is stretched tight. If you take an elastic band and stretch it out as far as it will go, it feels tight too.

If you think of the body as a big teeter totter, when one side goes down the other side goes up, right? Let's try something…stretch your right hand down to your right knee. Your right shoulder goes along for the ride and goes down too. What happens to your left shoulder? It goes up. Like a marionette puppet on strings. Everything is connected. (Picture #1)

It is the same for our front muscles and our back muscles. If we bend or flex forward our hip muscles shorten (knots) and the back muscles stretch (elastic band). So as one side of the body is flexing or shortening the other side is lengthening. If you sit a lot, which most of us do, your front hip muscles are getting shorter, and that means that your back-hip muscles are getting stretched. When muscles get stretched too far or pulled on too much from the front, they begin to get little micro-tears. Just like an elastic band: if you stretch it too far it will start to get little tears and eventually snap. Your back muscles will never snap but they can get very sore and swollen from all the micro-tears. When people complain about back pain and back tightness that tells me that it is getting pulled or stretched too far from the knotted front muscles. There are rare cases, like if you have been hit with a bat or a car, which could cause you pain in the place where it hurts. But seriously, normally pain equals a muscle imbalance, and it is more likely it is coming from the tight forward bending muscles. (Pictures #2a and #2b)

So, how do we fix this? It's easy! You stretch or lengthen the front muscles and the back muscles get some relief, or slack. The more you stretch the knots out, the less pulling on your back. Let's try this with your hand. Make a fist. The palm of your hand is flexing to close the fingers tight. What happens to the back of your hand? It gets stretched tight. What happens when you open up your fist and stretch your fingers out? The back of your hand isn't tight anymore. It is exactly the same for every joint in our bodies. If you bend a joint, the bending muscles shorten and the muscles on the opposite side lengthen. Our bodies are happiest or most comfortable when our muscles are balanced, and one side is not pulling harder than the other. For every action there is a reaction.

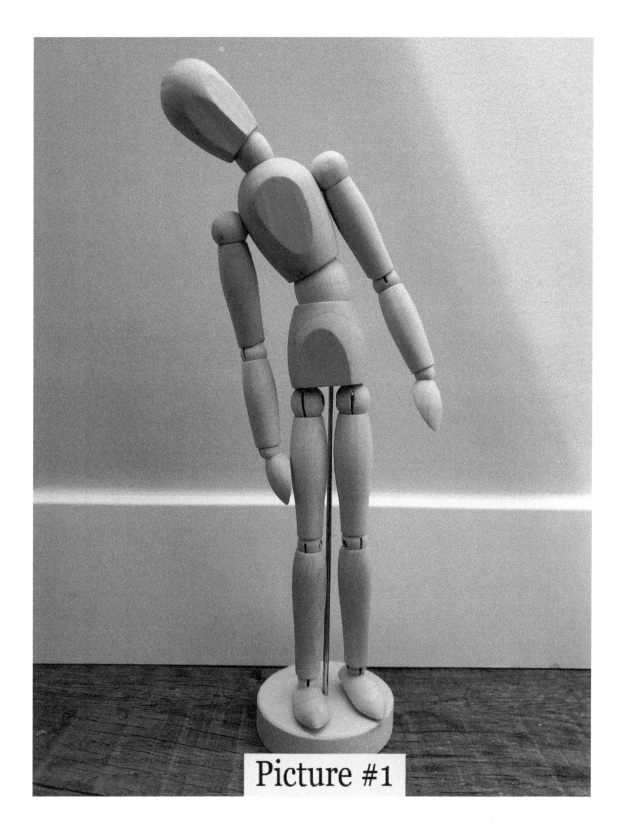

Picture #1

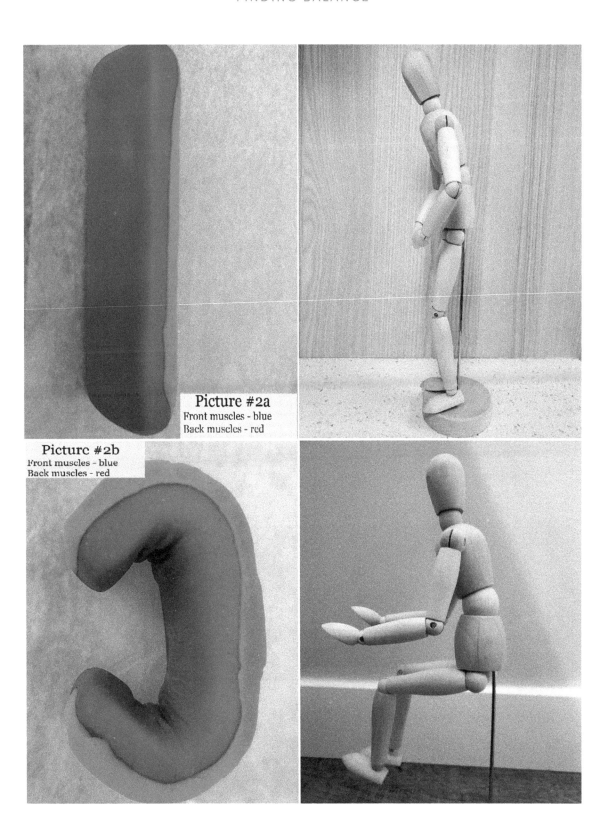

Picture #2a
Front muscles - blue
Back muscles - red

Picture #2b
Front muscles - blue
Back muscles - red

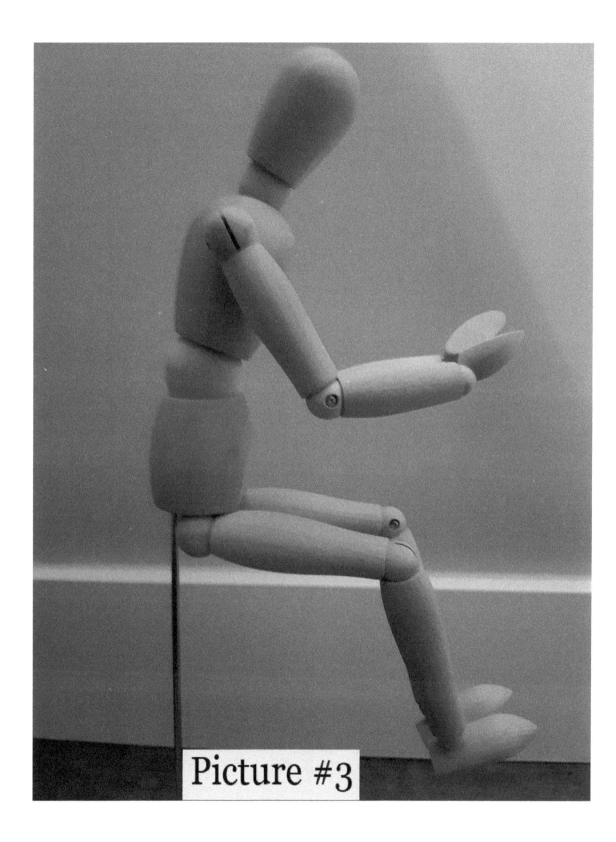

Picture #3

If you look down a lot of the time…say texting, reading, or typing, the front muscles of your neck will shorten and tighten. Over time these muscles will get shorter and shorter, pulling on the back of your neck. (Picture #3) This can cause pain, headaches and swelling in the back of your neck. The solution is to stretch the front muscles of your neck.

For some reason, we associate pain with that area being the problem. Pain is a problem, but the pain is a symptom of being stretched too far. Stretching the part of our body that hurts is really just making the stretched muscles longer. It feels good temporarily because you are giving it some relief. But then the tears get worse, and the front muscles have more room to shorten and create more of an imbalance.

Visual Examples:

- Pecs (short for, Pectoralis Major and Minor) and neck muscles tight, shoulders roll inwards – Blue.
  The shoulder blades get pulled into armpits, stretching the muscles between the shoulder blades and back of neck too long – Red.
  (Pictures #4 and #5)
- Anterior hips tight – Blue.
  Glutes and low back muscles get stretched too long – Red. (Picture #6)
- Quads and hips tight – Blue. Hamstrings stretched too long – Red. (Picture #7)

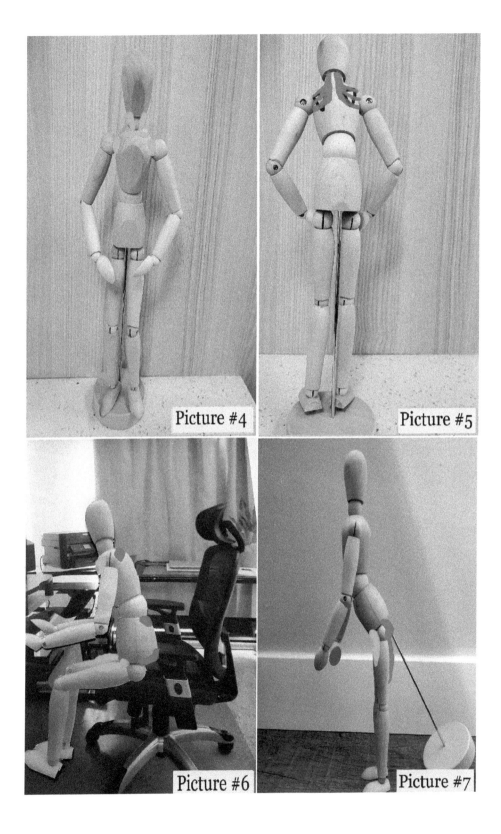

Picture #4

Picture #5

Picture #6

Picture #7

Let us get down to Business…

Sleeping – We spend a lot of our lives sleeping. It is good for us. It helps us heal and helps our minds focus. However, it also creates a large majority of our dysfunctions. Whether you are sitting or holding any position for a long period of time our muscles shorten where we bend, right? Right!

Sleeping positions add to our daytime habits. Typically, when you have short muscles, our body likes to keep them short for our comfort. If we have an injury our bodies like to protect that area by shortening the muscles in that area to give us comfort. Unfortunately, that is not the best thing for us. Short muscles getting shorter cause muscle imbalances and therefore dysfunction and eventually pain.

So, if you sleep primarily on one side, that shoulder, hip and neck on that side will become tighter. Body weight on a bent joint increases the folding of the muscles. Remember we have little spider web type adhesions forming all the time in our connective tissues, this can really add up over time and the fold can become solidified. (Pictures #8 and #9)

When we lie on our shoulder it curls inward towards the centre of our bodies. This makes the muscles bunch up or fold. It also shortens the pectoral muscles and Lat (short for, Latissimus Dorsi) muscle on that side - Blue. As a result of the shortening front muscles, and remembering we are just big teeter totters, the back muscles get stretched. The shoulder blade gets pulled into the armpit area and stretches the muscles between the shoulder blade and spine. This stretching in the back can cause little micro tears, swelling and pain over time. As one side shortens the opposite side lengthens. Our muscles only have so much give before they begin to tear. – Red. (Picture #10)

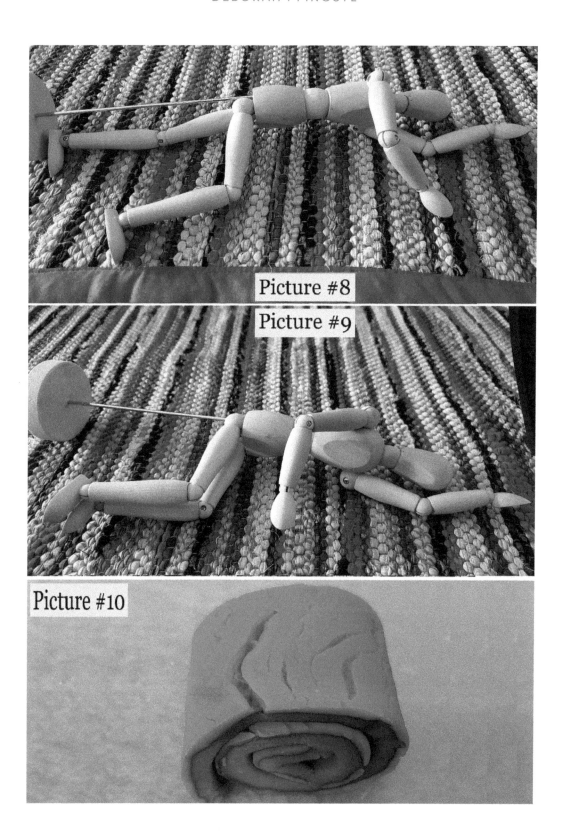

Picture #8

Picture #9

Picture #10

Unfortunately, we associate pain with knots or a problem where it hurts that needs to be worked out. That is not completely true… tearing, swelling and pain is a problem. What is causing the tearing is the real problem. By stretching the already lengthened back muscles we are causing more damage. It feels better temporarily, but it also gives more room for the front muscles to get shorter and create more imbalance.

How do we fix this? You cannot change the way you sleep, or at least it is extremely difficult to change the way you sleep. You can start off in a good position but ultimately our mind and body do whatever they want when we are sleeping. I tell my clients that sleep is more important than how you sleep. If sleeping on your head is how you sleep, then do it. Trying to change our bodies sleeping habits only messes up our sleep.

The best we can do is stretch out the knots during the day and ice where it hurts before bed. To correct the problem, we have to break up the adhesions to allow the shoulder to go back to a neutral position. Our tissue is very much like a piece of gum. When you chew gum, it becomes soft and stretches easily. When the gum is cold, and you try to stretch it out it will snap. Our tissue works the same way. Using the "Gum Rule", we only stretch when we are warm and never after we have iced. After we are done stretching, we ice the place that hurts for 20 mins. Once the front knotted muscles are worked out, we can start strengthening the stretched-out muscles and create balance.

- Pec Stretches (Pictures #11 and #12)

Stretches for Pecs with strengthening for Rhomboids (muscles between your shoulder blades). The stretch should feel good, not painful, in the front. Engage the back muscles to squeeze the shoulder blades together. Hold for 5 seconds.

Also, when sleeping our neck muscles shorten on the side we sleep on. Having a pillow between your shoulder and head will help to keep the neck muscles from shortening as well. (Lumbar pillow, tube, is good)

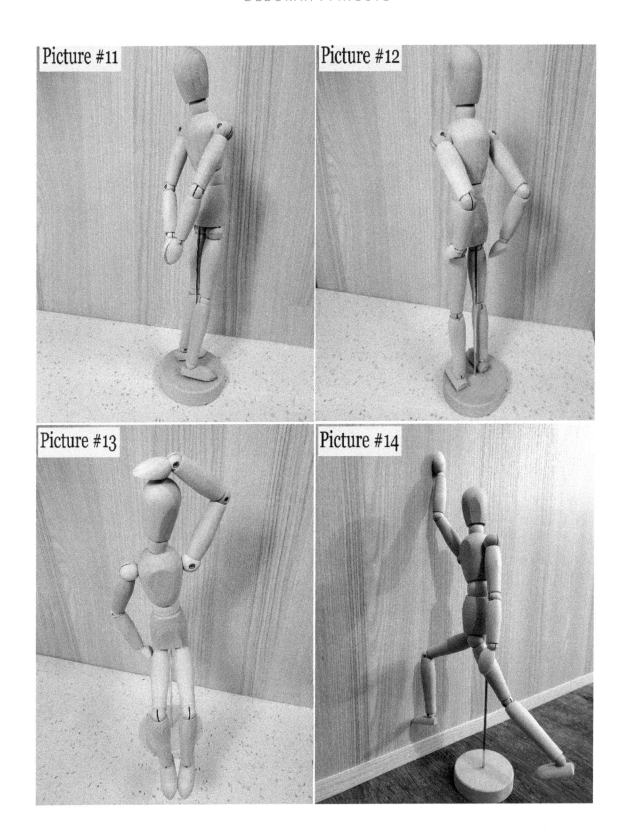

- Neck Stretch/Chair Stretch (Picture #13)

Place your hand under the seat of your chair on the side you are wanting to stretch. With your other hand, gently lay it on top of your head. Do not pull on your head. The stretch should feel good not painful. (Picture #13)

Leaning on your elbow – pushes your shoulder up into your ear. Folds or knots form in the space between your shoulder and neck. Do the Chair Stretch (Picture #13) for the neck.Stretches should be done slowly with about 30 seconds of hold time. Remember to breathe and relax as you are stretching. Never tug or bounce while you are stretching as this can cause more tears. Stretches should be done 2-3 times per day and not more. Muscle tissue, when you stretch it, does not stay stretched. Very much like raw pizza dough, it will spring back to where it was. This is why you need to stretch often and daily. More is not better. Make each stretch really count. Feel the place you are stretching. You should feel a good stretch and not pain. If it hurts, back off a bit. Feel the muscle lengthening… this is called the Ahhh factor, because it feels so good when the muscle releases. Everyone is different, so it may take you more or less than 30 seconds to get to the Ahhh factor. You can stretch a bit deeper if the muscles relax and allow it. Listen to your body. It will let you know when enough is enough.

- Lat Stretch (Picture #14)

Place the toe and knee against a wall on the side you want to stretch. The Lat muscle is a really long muscle that goes from your armpit to your low back. It is important to twist when doing a Lat stretch as the muscle is on an angle. Place your hand near the wall above your head. Don't lean in at this point. Twist your body and your head away from the wall, keeping your knee and toes on the wall as your anchor. Now lean in while in the twisted position. Remember to breathe and relax while stretching. Let your body "slunk" into the wall. Relaxing and resting as close to the wall as you can comfortably. Sticking your hip out like you are leaning on a lamp post. Enjoy the stretch for 30 full seconds.

- Anterior Neck Stretches – "Ugly Face" (Picture #15)

Holding Baby, Nursing and Hip Holding: We only bend one way, right… We are also looking down a lot while we are doing these actions, so the muscles in the front of our necks also get shortened (Blue), causing pain in the back of our neck (Red). Stretching the front of the neck is not as hard as it sounds. It is more than just looking up though. You place flat hands just below the collar bones. Press your hands inward towards your back and pull down at the same time. While doing that bring your chin up, do not tilt your head all the way back, just nose pointing to the ceiling. Also pull your lower lip up too. I call this making the "Ugly Face". Doing this in the shower with the warm water on the front of your neck feels great and helps the neck muscles to lengthen. Also no one can see you making the Ugly Face...

- Pregnancy Imbalances (Pictures #16a, #16b, #17a and #17b)
- Doorway Pec Stretch (Picture #18)

Nursing also requires you to hold and have incredible endurance for long periods of time. Although babies are adorable little bundles of love, they are also very heavy. This causes our pec muscles, shoulders, elbows and wrists to get short and tight (Blue - Pictures 16a and 16b). Repetitive strain is not only for repetitive movements but also for repetitive holding of muscles (Red - Pictures 17a and 17b). Our pec muscles and arms get tight. A good stretch for pecs is in the doorway (Picture #18). Make sure your arms come straight out from your shoulders with elbows bent at a 90-degree angle or the shape of an L. Lean through the doorway allowing the pecs to lengthen. Again, about 30 seconds. You can do a bit of a lunge position to support your back and body. Keep an eye on your shoulders as you lean through the doorway, making sure your arms are straight out from your shoulders. You can also incorporate a neck stretch as well if you want.

The "Ugly Face" Stretch

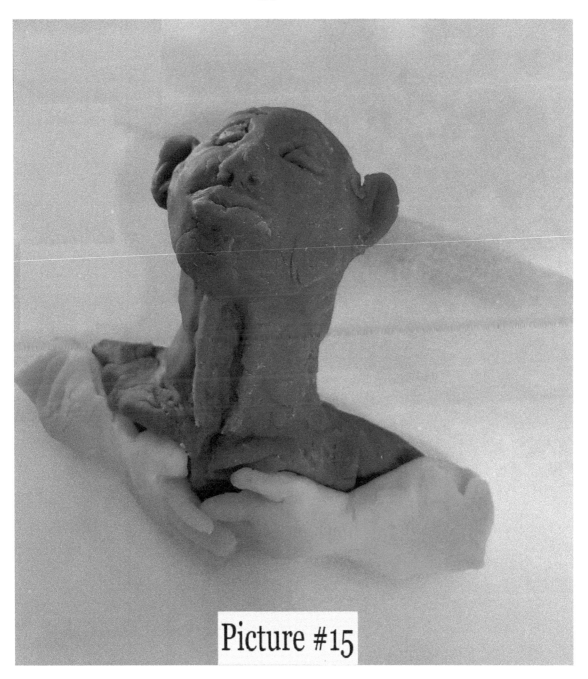

Picture #15

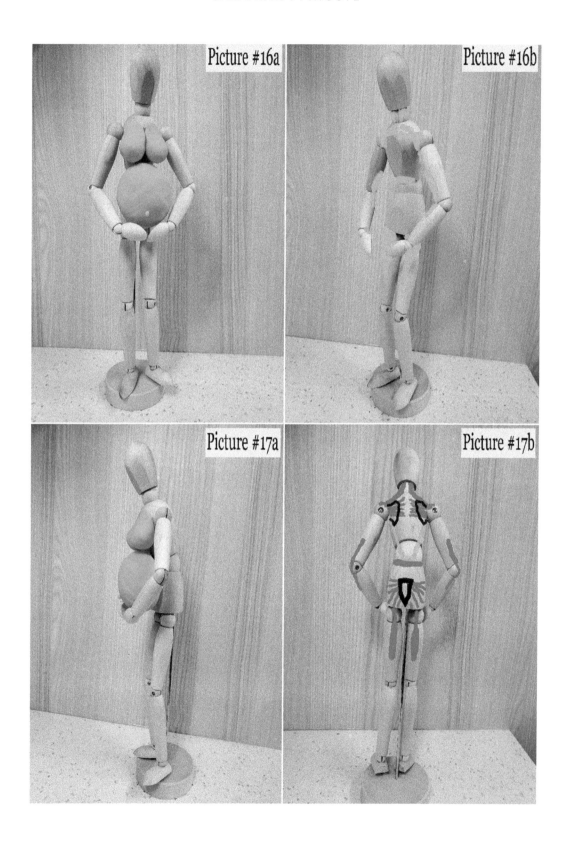

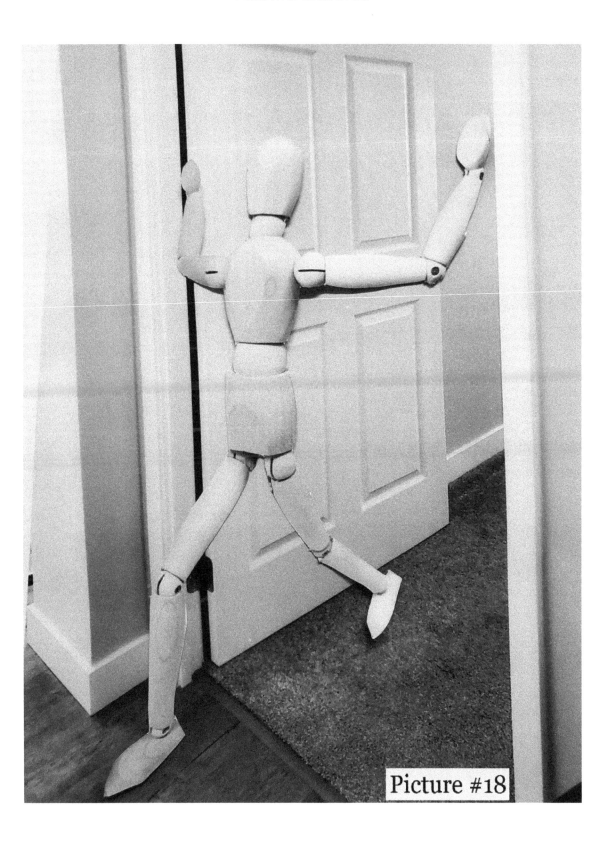

Picture #18

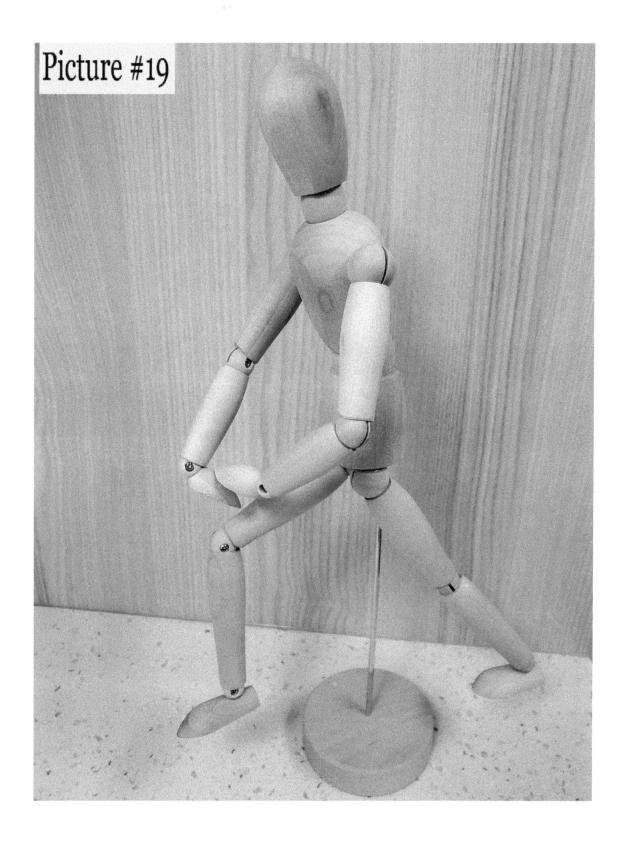

Picture #19

Larger babies we often hold on our hips while we are doing things with the other hand. Hip elevation and forearm tightness are the problem here. Forearm stretches are easy. Stand in front of your bed and place one hand flat on the bed with the fingers pointing towards the centre of your body. Again, a bit of a lunge position will help give your body support. Lean your body away from the bed to create an anglc so not to be directly over the hand. The elbow remains straight during the stretch. Your fingers on the arm you are stretching may curl up a bit. Place your other hand flat on the curled fingers to help keep them straight. Remember, never stretch to pain. If it is painful in a bad way ease off a bit. You can go a bit deeper when the muscles release into the Ahhh factor. Do this on the other arm too, 2-3 times a day. (Picture #19)

Hip elevation from resting your bundle of joy on it can cause hip or pelvis imbalances. A lunge stretch is a great way to help keep the hips balanced. Grab a cushion to place under your knee. The hip you are stretching will have the cushion under its knee. The opposite leg will take a big step forward, so that the stretching leg is on an angle backwards. Make sure the forward leg has the knee directly over the ankle during this stretch so not to hurt the bent knee. As you breathe and relax into this stretch your body should sink downward slightly. Lean back a bit to feel the stretch in the front of your hip. Hold this stretch 30 seconds while relaxing and sinking. It is good to place one hand on the forward bent knee to help with balance and leaning backwards. A gentle push on the knee increases the stretch to the front hip. The other hand can hold onto a stable nearby bed, couch or chair for balance.

- Lunge Stretch (Picture #20)

This lunge stretch is good for people who sit a lot as well. Stretch both sides to feel which side is tighter. Stretch the tighter side a bit more to help with muscle balancing.

If leaning backwards is too painful or difficult you can place your foot on a chair behind you and dip down, holding a chair or something stable in front of you. Another way to stretch the front of your hip is to lie on your back in bed with your buttock as close to the edge of the bed as possible. Hang your leg over the edge of the bed. Try to do this in a place that is high enough so that your foot does not touch the floor. Let gravity do the work for you. If your foot touches the floor, try placing a pillow under your buttock to give some elevation. You should feel a good pull in the front hip area, and not pain. If you find that your back is arching or it is too uncomfortable, move your body away from the edge of the bed to give your leg more support, but still allowing your leg to hang from the knee. As the stretch becomes easier, move closer to the edge of the bed again. Using heat to relax the front hip muscles is also a good idea. Warm, not hot heat, for 5 to 10 minutes is enough.

If this is still too uncomfortable for you try lying on a ball about the size of a tennis ball. Make sure it is not too hard. Or you can use a foam roller. You can rest the ball or foam roller in the spot that is tight in the front of your hip. You will know when you are on it! Hold this stretch for 30 seconds or until the Ahhh factor. Move ball or foam roller to the next tight spot in the same hip and repeat until all the tightness is out. It is okay to heat the area first but **not** ice first. Ice is for after stretching. A Quad Stretch is also good for stretching the front of the hip. Please do not do this one if you are pregnant, as you could lose your balance and fall.

- Quad Stretch (Picture #21)

SI joint or sacroiliac joint is in your low back near your tailbone. It is the place where your sacrum (the triangle at the base of your spine) and ilium (or pelvis) form a hinge joint. Much like a door hinge this joint is very thin and not as stable as the ball and socket joints of the hips and shoulders. When our hip bones are unbalanced, it can cause rubbing and damage to this joint. The rubbing can cause swelling which can lead to spasms. Sitting crossing our legs, resting one foot on the other knee in a number 4 position, sitting on the floor with knees bent and feet crossed (some call it crisscross apple sauce), sitting on your foot or even pregnancy can cause the SI joint to become damaged. Any sitting position where the knee is pointing away from your body can irritate the SI joint.

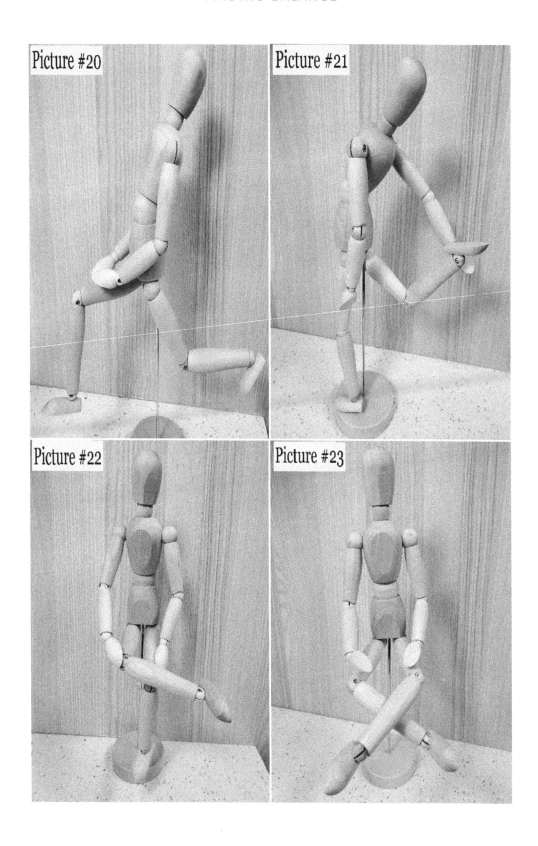

Picture #20

Picture #21

Picture #22

Picture #23

- SI Joint "No-No's" (Pictures #22 and #23)

Typically swelling caused by the rubbing in the SI joint can create spasms that normally run down the inside of the leg to the knee and even down to the foot. Spasms cause the muscles to shorten. This puts pressure on the medial knee, or part of the knee that faces inward towards the other knee. In turn the knee becomes imbalanced and swelling in the knee joint can occur. The spasm can travel down the calf as well pulling the foot inwards and upwards, this is called Supination.

The first key to helping the SI joint balance is to get rid of the swelling by icing the SI joint area. Once the swelling is reduced, you can begin some gentle stretches. Icing for two to three days in a row should be enough to help reduce the swelling. (See Chapter 6 for proper icing instructions)

Then warm, gentle stretches of the muscles running up the inside of the leg or "Adductors" is the next most important action to help balance the SI joint.

Of course, stopping the action that is causing this imbalance, like crossing legs, is also a good start. Pregnancy, unfortunately, is a tougher one as the forward weight and the hormones that cause the tendons to relax make the SI joint more vulnerable. Sorry Moms. Sometimes if the swelling of the joint gets too bad it can cause the glute or buttock muscles to spasm and pinch the Sciatic nerve that runs through them, causing more difficulties. Number 1 get the swelling out by icing the SI joint area. Number 2 gentle stretches when warm. Number 3 change what position(s) you sit in to help the muscles balance the SI joint again.

A good stretch to help the SI joint is the side stretch for the inside of your legs. Lean your body up against a wall to keep you straight and so your butt won't stick out. Separate your feet so that your stance is wider than your hips. Bend one knee, keeping your back against the wall. This stretches the other leg on the inside muscles. Do this stretch for both sides. Hold until you feel the Ahhh factor. As this gets easier, increase the distance between your feet to increase the stretch. (Picture #24)

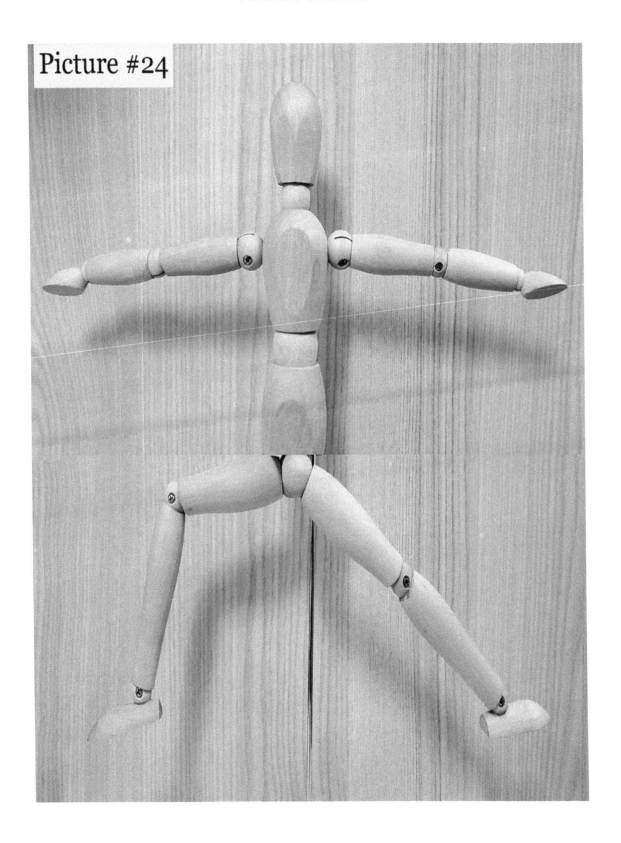

Picture #24

Chapter Five

"The Hairy Eyeball"

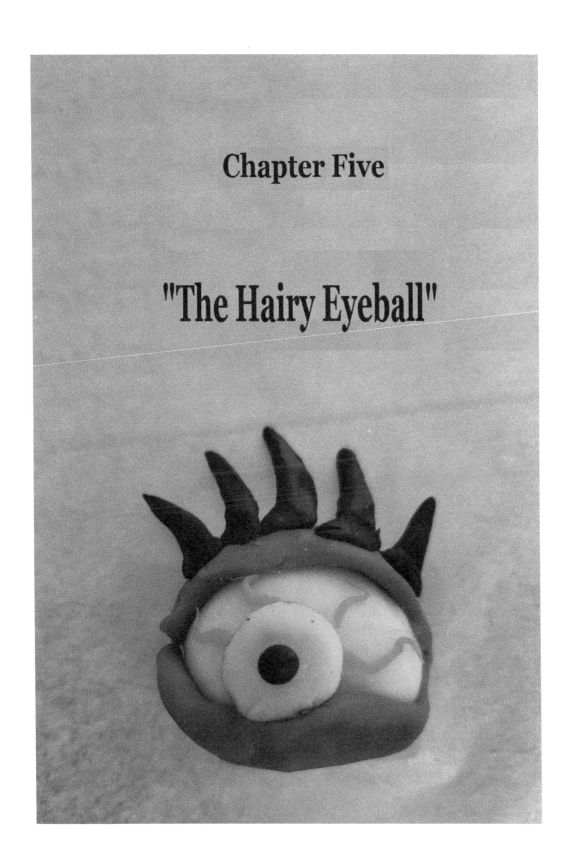

Going back to the beginning a bit… when I was working in the personal care homes, the health care aids would lie the residents down in the most comfortable position, on their backs. I worked mainly on their front muscles and noticed their back pain would disappear or dissipate without touching it. That's because their shoulders and hips were too tight, right!? As I worked on the tight front muscles, the stretched back muscles were getting relief. Now you see what I am talking about.

As I carried forward with my massage therapy practice and began getting more into the clinical side, I began working with people who were still in the work force and physically able to do most things.

So, here's the Scoop. Massage therapy is considered a comfort treatment by most people to this day. And that's okay. Yes, there are massages and massage therapists whose sole purpose is to give you comfort from your pain, like Mom did when we were children. If our backs or tummies hurt, she rubbed them. As a result, I feel that we associate pain with the place we need to rub. You hit your knee (ouch!) you rub your knee…pain goes away, right? Well, sometimes…

The question I want to ask you is: do you want temporary comfort or a solution to the problem? If it is a chronic or on-going pain problem, you probably want it to go away and not keep coming back. I know, silly question! Just rubbing the back is not going to cut it for a permanent solution. So, applying my lessons I had learned in the personal care homes, I stared getting people to lie down on their backs, not on their stomachs as they were used to for massage. Some looked at me, like are you sure…? I'd smile and nod yes. Some wouldn't question it, and some would lie on their stomachs anyway. I would just ask them to turn over onto their backs before we began. Now this is where it got interesting!

I will never forget the first time I got the "Hairy Eyeball." I had just finished transitioning from personal care to clinical work. A young lady came in for a massage with pain in the back of her neck and down into her shoulder blade on the right side. After I assessed her, I asked her to lie down on her back, facing upwards. She gave me the "are you sure" look, and then repeated that her pain was in the back. I smiled and nodded 'yes.' Reluctantly she laid on her back. As I lifted her right arm and started working on the front of her shoulder and into the armpit, I could see she was getting more and more annoyed. I asked her if the pressure was too much? "No", she replied. Continuing with the releasing of the front muscles I could see she was really getting worked up and bits of steam were coming out of her ears. Finally, she looked right at me and it happened. With utter frustration and irritation, she shot me the hairy eyeball. "Why are you working on my armpit when my back hurts?" she questioned with intense frustration.

I smiled at her and explained how the tight muscles in her armpit and shoulder were pulling on her neck and upper back. She did not seem convinced until it was time to turn over and *finally* get to her back. I started working on her neck and upper back, and she said with total surprise, "It doesn't hurt anymore!" like I might actually know what I am doing! The first 45 minutes of the one-hour massage took everything in my power to stick to my guns and not give in to her requests. The last 15 minutes of the treatment we laughed and joked. She was so happy by the end of the treatment. She came back again and again and sent her friends and family to see me. Each time she had a massage with me after that we had a good laugh about it.

My second hairy eyeball came into the clinic a short while after, with low back pain on the left side. I assessed him and asked him to lie on his back. Again… the "are you sure you want me to lie on my back" look. I smiled and nodded 'yes.' Reluctantly he laid on his back. During my assessment I felt his hips and realized that his front right hip was very tight. I asked him his profession and he said professional piano player. He was from out of town and could not wait to get back home before getting a massage. As I began working on the front of his right hip, he began telling me that the massage therapists where he is from (Ontario) were some of the best in Canada! He went on and on about their quality and amount of training they have. As I worked, I secretly smiled. After about 45 minutes went by, and he was getting more and more adamant about my lack of understanding, the steam from his ears was visible now. Then it happened! The hairy eyeball came out. "Okay, time to turn over," I said. I could see he was not impressed that I had wasted 55 minutes of an hour on the front of his hip, on the wrong side no less! As he turned over for the last 5 minutes of the treatment he said, "that didn't hurt to turn over!" I said nothing. Just a little smile on my face. He was shocked and overjoyed that his pain had disappeared, and I hadn't even touched his back. He asked for my business card so he could refer the entire band he was playing with. I said, "Sure (with a cheeky smile), and I didn't even study in Ontario." He gave me a nod and a grin and shook my hand.

CHAPTER SIX

Heat or Ice?

L et's talk about frozen peas.

They really are the best for therapy. They are small and round so they break up really well and conform to any shape for maximum surface coverage. Frozen peas can hold enough cold to ice effectively up to one hour in total before you have to put them back in the freezer. Frozen peas are guaranteed to get you numb after 20 minutes of icing. This way you can ice up to three spots, 20 minutes each before you have to put them back in the freezer. Why is it important to get numb when you are icing?

There are four levels you need to go through when icing properly (CBAN)

C – cold

B - burning

A - aching

N - numb

It is important you go through all of these stages when icing because the blood vessels close after 20 minutes in the numb stage. When blood vessels close, they create a vacuum like effect as they open. Blood vessels are perforated and that is what allows the fluid in the tissues to move in and out as they open and close. We need the blood vessels to close so that the fluid in our tissues can be sucked back into the blood vessel. If the blood vessel does not close all the way, you won't get the vacuum effect. If you only ice for 10 or 15 minutes, the blood vessel will not close all the way and it will take you longer to reduce the inflammation and therefore the pain.

When blood vessels are warm, they dilate, and the walls of the blood vessel stretch. The little holes or perforations allow the fluid to leak out into the surrounding tissues to create swelling. When the blood vessel is cold it constricts and gets tighter and narrower. It eventually closes completely after 20 minutes of icing, so it is important to take the frozen peas off. You don't want to restrict the blood flow too long or cause damage to the surrounding nerves. As the blood circulation returns to the area the blood vessels begin to warm up slowly and open again. The body itself is a vacuum. As the blood vessel opens it draws the fluid or edema back in. Try opening a plastic bag under water, it's the same principle.

The process of the blood vessel warming and opening and pulling edema back into the blood stream takes about an hour after you remove the peas. Let it warm up naturally. Don't rub the area or do any stretches while your tissue is cold. The iced tissue is more fragile and can become damaged easily. Imagine your tissues are like a piece of gum. Let's say you take your gum out of your mouth and let it get cold. What happens when you try to stretch cold gum? It breaks, right? It becomes easier to stretch when you chew on it and warm it up again. Our tissues are just like gum. When we are cold, we can cause damage to our tissues if we stretch them. Our tissues are more pliable when warm and less susceptible to injury.

Some ice packs are hard and square, so they don't give you maximum coverage. Gel packs rarely stay cold enough to get you numb and they are a one-shot deal before they have to go back into the freezer. Peas can be used in three places for 20 minutes each before they have to go back in the freezer. Peas are cheap and you can use them over and over. Every home should have a therapeutic bag of peas. Remember, cheap peas work just as good as the expensive peas. Keep your bag of therapeutic peas separate so you don't eat them, they will still be there when you need them.

Why not corn or mixed vegetables? Well corn sticks together too much and does not break up well. The carrots in the mixed veggies thaw faster and will go soft making the mixture stick together and get lumpy. But if that is all you have and you need to ice, go for it! I have used frozen sausages in a pinch. Hey, whatever works. The idea is to get numb though and alcohol does not count.

Always remember to wrap your frozen peas in a thin tea towel or something not too thick. One layer of cloth should be between you and your peas to protect your skin from getting damaged. Also, remember to time it. Twenty minutes only, no more, no less. More is not better as the blood vessel is already closed. Less than 20 minutes and the blood vessel will not close all the way and you won't get the vacuum effect.

Heat is to be used when no swelling is present.

There are three levels of injury.

Acute injury is typically the first two to three days after the injury happens. This is strictly the R.I.C.E. stage. Rest, Ice, Compression, and Elevation. It depends on how severe the injury is. A sprain will take a week sometimes to get past the acute stage. A tear can take much longer to heal. See your family doctor or nearby clinic to determine which it is.

Sub-acute is the second stage and a combination of heat and ice, in that order, is recommended. You should be ready to incorporate some gentle stretches to assist the healing process at this point. Remember the "Gum Rule", only stretch when you are warm. Ice is last and is always 20 minutes. Remember to wait an hour after icing before you apply heat or stretch. Icing before bed can also help you sleep more comfortably.

Chronic is the last stage. This happens when the injury persists for more than six months. If there is still inflammation at this point you need to see your doctor. If no swelling is present, use heat to relax and ease the stiffness. There is most likely scar tissue, and it does not stretch as well as muscle tissue. Heat is a good way to help scar tissue to stretch.

If you are uncertain if swelling is present, Ice. Both heat and ice bring blood to the area, but heat opens the blood vessels and cold closes them. Once the heat or ice is removed the area will become red with blood circulation. If swelling is present and you place heat on it, more fluid will be allowed to drain out of the blood vessel into the tissues and you will feel stiffer the next day. It feels good to heat sometimes but it can be temporary relief. Icing when unsure guarantees you will not get more swelling and pain. Frozen peas are drug-free and are an effective tool for pain relief.

Let's talk about stretches. It is okay to research general stretches. For instance, pectoral muscles or hip flexor muscles. But when the issue is more localized you need to consult a professional (and not the internet) to get the exact stretches you need to target the place you are needing to stretch. Just remember that where you feel the pain is most likely not the place that needs to stretch.

CONCLUSION

At this point I would like to say that these are strictly my opinions and observations over the last eighteen plus years of practice. I realize some will have very strong opposing views. That is human nature. I am not saying that this is the best way to practice massage therapy, just simply the way I practice massage therapy. There is more than one correct way to help someone heal.

I would also like to say that it does frustrate me to see clients receiving treatment without improvements. They will continue to go to the same therapist, doctor, chiropractor…and keep getting the same result each time, temporary relief. In my opinion, if you are receiving therapy and if after six treatments you are not seeing or feeling obvious changes, it is time to find something else. Not everyone benefits from the same treatment. We are made up of the exact same elements, number of bones, muscles and tissues for the majority. But we are **all** completely unique in our makeup. What works for one may not work for another. Whether it is massage, chiropractic, acupuncture, energy work or physiotherapy… I always tell my clients that if it works, do it. And if it doesn't work, try something else.

I personally want my clients to get to a point where they don't need me anymore. They are educated enough to go it alone and maintain their bodies and injuries by themselves. That is, and always will be my goal. I realize I am not a perfect therapist and that I am still continuously learning. All being well I hope to continue working as a massage therapist for the next fifteen years. I know I will learn much more in that time.

FOR A LAUGH

One client asked me, completely innocently, if my massage therapy book would have a "Happy Ending." I laughed, and she looked at me with confused eyes. I explained the connotation, and we both had a good laugh!

Another client asked me what the title of my book would be. I told her I hadn't decided yet. She suggested I call it "Shut up and let me do my job and you will feel better!" I almost fell off my stool laughing but decided against naming it that.

This book was partially written during the Covid-19 pandemic. Some time to think and laugh with my partner while isolated resulted in a possible title being: "Rub in the Time of Covid" as in the novel, "Love in the Time of Cholera," by Gabriel García Márquez.

Song titles for which we substituted the word "rub" for "love" are:

- "What about Rub" by Heart – my personal favorite
- "Addicted to Rub" by Robert Palmer
- "You Give Rub a Bad Name" by Bon Jovi
- "You Can't Hurry Rub" by Phil Collins
- "What's Rub Got to Do with It" by Tina Turner
- "All You Need is Rub" by The Beatles
- And for the days when I am all used-up energy wise: "I'm All out of Rub" by Air Supply

THE END

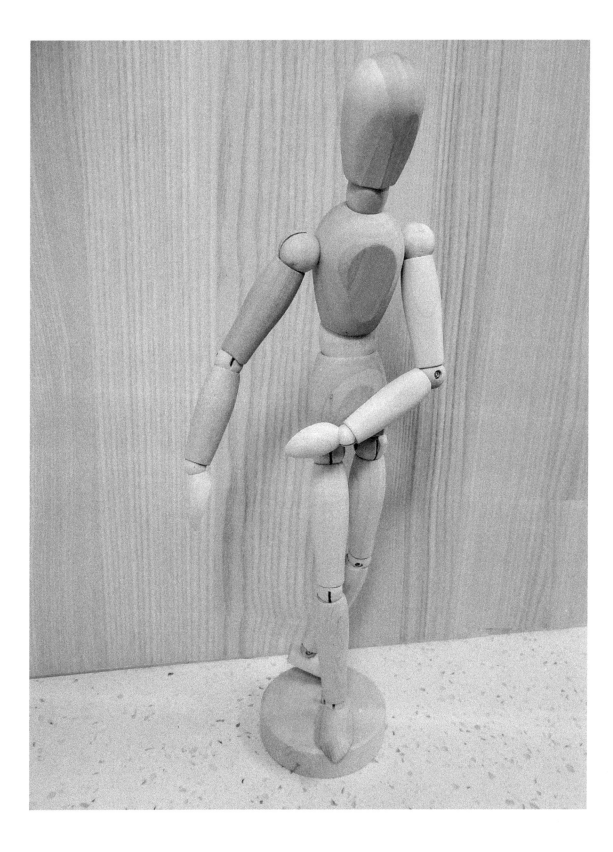

ACKNOWLEDGEMENTS

I would like to extend my gratitude to the following people for their patience, guidance and friendship.

Melva McLean - Editor
Chris Gonske - Interior Photo Set Up
Erna Wiebe - Exterior Photos
S. Ross Wiebe - Teeter Totter Creation
Jeff and Joanna Quail - Test Readers
Leanne Bochinski - Test Reader
Theresa and David Ronson - Test Readers
Libby Powell - Test Reader

CPSIA information can be obtained
at www.ICGtesting.com
Printed in the USA
BVHW021014071221
622674BV00009B/5